Surface & Radiological ANATOMY

THIRD EDITION

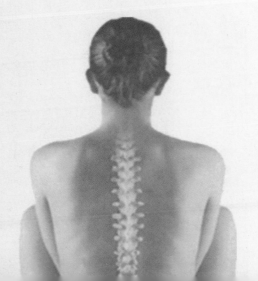

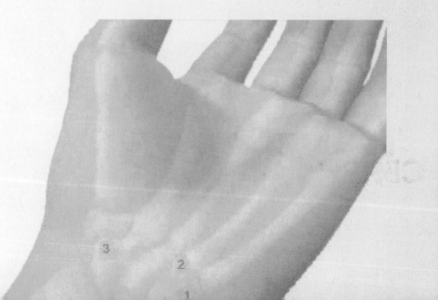

Surface and Radiological ANATOMY

THIRD EDITION

A. Halim MBBS MS FIMSA

Ex-head and Professor of Anatomy
King George's Medical College
Lucknow University

WHO Fellow in Medical Education (UK)
Fellow British Association of Clinical Anatomists

Ex-member Academic Council, King George's
Medical and Dental Universities

Lucknow, India

CBS

CBS Publishers & Distributors Pvt Ltd

New Delhi • Bengaluru • Pune • Kochi • Chennai

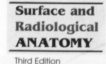

Surface and Radiological ANATOMY

Third Edition

ISBN: 978-81-239-1952-2

Copyright © Author and Publishers

Third Edition: 2011
First Edition: 1988
Second Edition: 1993

Published by Satish Kumar Jain and produced by Vinod K. Jain for
CBS Publishers & Distributors Pvt Ltd
4819/XI Prahlad Street, 24 Ansari Road, Daryaganj, New Delhi 110 002, India.
Ph: 011-23289259, 011-23266861/67   Fax: 011-23243014   Website: www.cbspd.com
                                                                  e-mail: delhi@cbspd.com
                                                                  cbspubs@vsnl.com
                                                                  cbspubs@airtelmail.in

Branches

• Bengaluru: Seema House 2975, 17th Cross, K.R. Road,
  Banasankari 2nd Stage, Bengaluru 560 070, Karnataka
  Ph: 080-26771678/79   Fax: 080-26771680   e-mail: bangalore@cbspd.com

• Pune: Bhuruk Prestige, Sr. No. 52/12/2+1+3/2 Narhe, Haveli
  (Near Katraj-Dehu Road Bypass), Pune 411 051, Maharashtra
  Ph: 020-64704058, 64704059   Fax: 020-24300160   e-mail: pune@cbspd.com

• Kochi: 36/14 Kalluvilakam, Lissie Hospital Road, Kochi 682 018, Kerala
  Ph: 0484-4059061-65   Fax: 0484-4059065   e-mail: cochin@cbspd.com

• Chennai: 20, West Park Road, Shenoy Nagar, Chennai 600 030, Tamil Nadu
  Ph: 044-26260666, 26208620   Fax: 044-45530020   email: chennai@cbspd.com

Printed at Paras Offset Pvt. Ltd., C-176, Naraina Industrial Area Phase-I, New Delhi

to
my students

"A teacher affects eternity,
he can never tell where his influence stops"

—Henry Brooks Adams

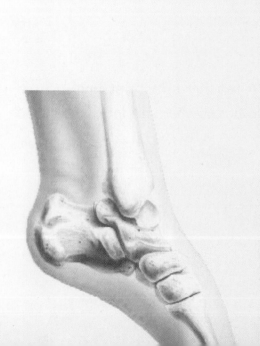

Preface to the Third Edition

In preparing the third edition of this book which has been well received for almost over two decades, I have retained the earlier version for its easy approach to the subject. The diagrams of surface anatomy in Part I have been coloured since colour captures a reality that is more consistent with the mode of learning and has become an increasingly important element for most of the students today. Apart from this, instead of abbreviated labelling full labelling of the figures has been done for better understanding.

In Part II the radiographs by repeated printing had become indistinct and have been mostly replaced by photographs of digital X-ray plates for their clarity. New ultrasonographs, computerised axial tomographs and MRI photographs have been put in.

The new imaging techniques have replaced contrast radiographic techniques like bronchography and cholecystography. Ultrasonography of hepatobiliary system, for example, is more sensitive than cholecystography in detecting small stones and biliary sludge and moreover the patients are not exposed to radiation. Contrast radiographs have their anatomical value to the student so chapters dealing with these have been retained.

I hope that the changes which have been made will facilitate the understanding of the text.

A. Halim

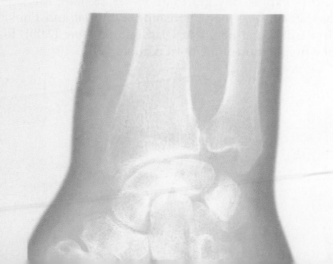

Acknowledgements

I wish to acknowledge my thanks to many of my colleagues whose criticism and advice guided me in preparing this book. I am grateful to Prof GN Agarwal, Head of the Department of Radiology, King George's Medical College, Lucknow, who very kindly provided most of the radiographs. The radiographs in the chapter on bone age estimation and ossification of limb bones were acquired from the department of anatomy, King George's Medical College and were due to research work done by Prof Mahadi Hasan and Prof ID Bajaj for their MS theses. I am thankful to them for allowing me to use these radiographs in my book.

I wish to express my appreciation of the many laborious hours spent by the artist Mr GC Das for successfully executing the illustrations and for carefully reproducing the tracings of the radiographs. The photographic prints were made by Mr VP Srivastava, Chief Technical Officer, Central Photographic Section, King George's Medical College, Lucknow. I am thankful to Mr RS Saxena, of the Department of Anatomy, KGMC, for the careful typing and retyping of the script.

I will be failing badly if I do not mention the encouragement which I received from my wife and my children in writing the book which has been a unique experience for the preparation of this edition.

For this revised edition I am most grateful to Dr Ratan Kumar Singh of Charak Diagnostic and Research Centre, Lucknow, for providing me digital radiographs. I am much indebted to Prof Ragini Singh, Head Department of Radiodiagnosis, and Prof Naseem Jamal, Department of Radiotherapy, CSM Medical University, for giving me CT photographs and USG strips.

I wish to thank Mr Ravi Kapoor, a famous photographer of Lucknow, for preparing photographic prints of the new radiographs. I also extend my most sincere appreciate to Mr Majumdar, the artist, for his careful tracings of the new radiographs.

Finally, I wish to express my gratitude to Mr SK Jain, Managing Director, Mr YN Arjuna, Senior Director—Publishing, Editorial and Publicity, and the editorial staff of CBS Publishers and Distributors, New Delhi, for their great assistance in the preparation of the third edition.

A. Halim

Preface to the First Edition

Surface and radiological anatomy form an important subdivision of anatomy. When a patient is examined it is his anatomy which is being examined. **Surface anatomy** is the study of deeper parts in relation to the skin surface. A mental picture of surface anatomy is needed by every doctor during the physical examination of a case whether it is by inspection, palpation, percussion or auscultation.

Radiological anatomy is the study of deeper organs by plain or contrast radiography. Diagnostic radiology is one of the most widely used investigation. Knowledge of the normal radiological appearances is indispensable as a background for the proper interpretation of radiographs for clinical purposes.

There has been a pressing need for a handy book on surface and radiological anatomy for students preparing for their examinations in this basic medical subject, hence this humble attempt on my part. Each statement included in this book has been drawn from the best known anatomy, radiology, medicine and surgery textbooks to make it authentic.

The book has been arranged in two sections. In the first section on surface anatomy it has been my endeavour to give in a systematic manner the marks which have to be put in outlining a particular structure so that the student does not have to search out the surface projection data from continuously written paragraphs as is usual in other books available on the subject. The structures intended for surface marking have been arranged in alphabetical order in subsections on arteries, veins, nerves, glands, viscera, joints, etc. to make them easy for reference.

The second section deals with radiological anatomy. The value of X-rays for the study of anatomy need not be stressed. It has been the aim to organise and to set down as concisely as possible what are considered basic facts of normal radiographic anatomy. Radiographs of different regions of the body in standard positions have been given with well elucidated parallel line diagrams and elaborate descriptions. The third chapter in this section has been specially written for the purpose of bone age estimation. Line diagrams depicting the sequence of ossification of union in different regions have been specially prepared to help student in assessing the bone age. A large number of radiographs of different age groups have been added to give the student an exercise on age determination on the basis of sequence of ossification and union in that region. Three tables to help the student better have been compiled.

Techniques of radiological procedures are described particularly those dealing with the more complicated diagnostic procedures such as bronchography.

The care of the subject before and after such investigations has also been given as the student should have some idea of what the examination entails and the way it is conducted.

There is a separate chapter on angiography which is one of the more specialised area of diagnostic radiology. Aortography and cerebral angiography has been dealt with in some detail. Some of the more advanced techniques are out of the scope of this elementary book and hence have been left out.

At the end a chapter on the new imaging devices has been added to give the student some idea of these body-scanning techniques which have revolutionised diagnostic medicine in the past two decades.

A. Halim

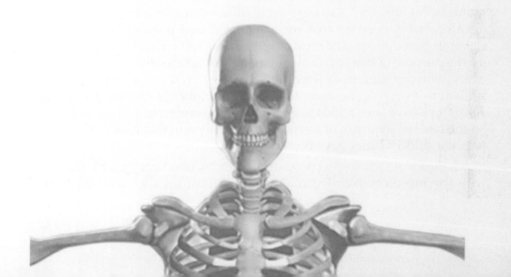

Contents

Part I: SURFACE ANATOMY

Part II: RADIOLOGICAL ANATOMY

Part I
Surface Anatomy

 SUPERIOR EXTREMITY

 INFERIOR EXTREMITY

 THORAX

 ABDOMEN AND PELVIS

 HEAD AND NECK

 BRAIN

NOTES

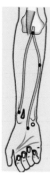# Introduction

The surface anatomy deals with the study of position of structures in relationship to the skin surface of the body. It helps in exploring these structures from the surface wherever necessary. Bony, muscular and other landmarks on the surface of the body are taken as guides. The landmarks may be visible or palpable.

1. *Visible landmarks* can be seen on inspection as they produce irregularities in the surface outline of the body. Majority of them are produced by bones or cartilages. Nipple and umbilicus also fall in this category.
2. *Palpable landmarks* are felt through the skin. Muscles and tendons become palpable by being put into contraction, arteries by their pulsations and nerves by rolling against bones. Spermatic cord and parotid duct can also be felt through the skin.

Important visible and palpable landmarks have been described and indicated in diagrams. While drawing the surface marking of a particular structure, the student is advised to put the required points first and then to join these by various lines as instructed.

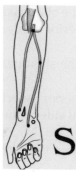

Superior Extremity

 ## SHOULDER, AXILLA, ARM AND ELBOW REGIONS

SURFACE LANDMARKS (Anterior Aspect) (Fig. 1.1)

- **Anterior axillary fold** is formed by the rounded lower border of pectoralis major. It becomes prominent when the abducted arm is adducted against resistance.
- **Clavicular head of pectoralis major** can be recognised as it contracts when the arm is flexed to a right angle.
- **Coracoid process** points almost straight forward, 2.5 cm vertically below the junction of the lateral fourth and medial three-fourths of the clavicle. Anterior fibres of deltoid cover it.

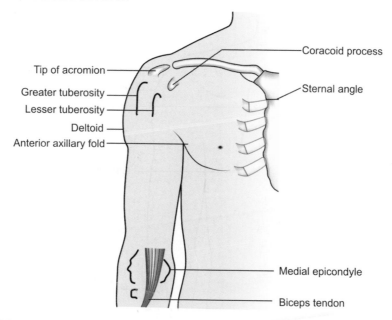

Tip of acromion
Greater tuberosity
Lesser tuberosity
Deltoid
Anterior axillary fold

Coracoid process
Sternal angle

Medial epicondyle
Biceps tendon

Fig. 1.1: Surface landmarks—shoulder, axilla, arm and elbow regions (anterior aspect)

- **Deltoid insertion** can be identified when the arm is maintained in the abducted position. It is half a way down the lateral aspect of humerus. Its anterior border can also be easily seen.
- **Greater tuberosity of humerus** is the most lateral bony point in the shoulder region.
- **Lateral epicondyle of humerus** is readily recognisable from the posterior aspect in the upper part of a well marked depression situated on the lateral side of the middle line.
- **Lesser tuberosity of humerus** lies 3 cm below the tip of the acromion on the anterior aspect of the shoulder.
- **Medial epicondyle of humerous** is a conspicuous landmark felt easily on the medial side in a flexed elbow.
- **Sternal angle (angle of Louis)** can be easily felt as a ridge by running the finger downwards on the sternum from the suprasternal notch. Traced laterally it leads to second costal cartilage. The ribs can be counted downwards after the second rib has been located.
- **Tendon of biceps** becomes prominent when the elbow is flexed, it can be grasped in the cubital fossa.
- **Tip of acromion** is situated lateral to the acromioclavicular joint and can be easily felt.

SURFACE LANDMARKS (Posterior Aspect) (Fig. 1.2)

- **Acromial angle:** Lower border of the crest of the spine becomes continues with the lateral border of the acromion at this angle.

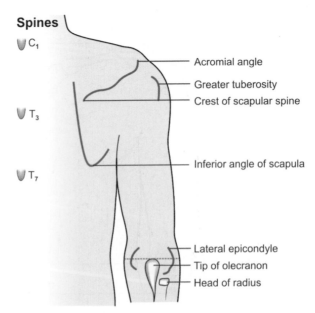

Fig. 1.2: Surface landmarks—shoulder, axilla, arm and elbow regions (posterior aspect)

- **Apex of the olecranon** can be felt well to the inner side of the mid-point of the inter-epicondylar line in an extended elbow. The tip of the olecranon and the two epicondyles form an isosceles triangle when the elbow is flexed.
- **Crest of the scapular spine** is subcutaneous throughout. It runs downwards and medially to reach the medial border of the bone opposite the third thoracic spine.
- **Head of the radius** is situated below the lateral epicondyle in the depression described above, 'lying in the valley behind the supinator longus (biceps)' (Holden). It can be felt to rotate when the forearm is alternately pronated and supinated.
- **Inferior angle of scapula** can be felt at the level of the seventh thoracic spine when the medial border of scapula is traced downwards.
- **Posterior surface of the olecranon** is subcutaneous and tapers from above downwards.
- **Triceps, lateral head** lies parallel to the posterior border of the deltoid. To its medial side is the long head of triceps.

SURFACE MARKINGS

Gland

Breast (Fig. 1.3)

- Put a mark at the margin of the sternum opposite the sternal angle.
- Mark the sternal end of the sixth costal cartilage.
- Draw the midaxillary line.

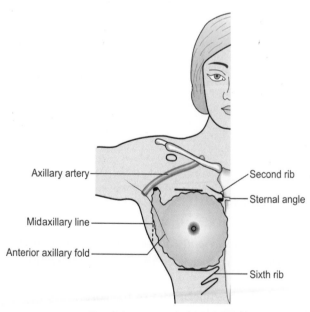

Fig. 1.3: Breast and axillary artery

- Put a mark on the pulsation of the axillary artery under cover of anterior axillary fold.
- Mark the second rib and cartilage.

The breast can now be indicated by drawing a circular line passing through these various points but going upwards into the axilla up to the axillary vessels to mark the tail of Spence.

JOINTS

The Elbow Joint

On the front the plane of the joint can be represented as follows (Fig. 1.4a).
- Put a point 2 cm below the medial epicondyle.
- Mark a point 2 cm below the lateral epicondyle.

Join these points by a line directed downwards and medially. The line is oblique because of the carrying angle and also represents the distal limit of the cavity of the joint.

The proximal limit of the joint cavity can be represented on the front of the arm by the following line (Fig. 1.4b).
- Put a point just above the tubercle on the coronoid process.
- Mark a point over the most lateral part of the front of the medial epicondyle.
- Mark the level of the head of the radius.
- Draw a curved line from the first point arching across to the last point

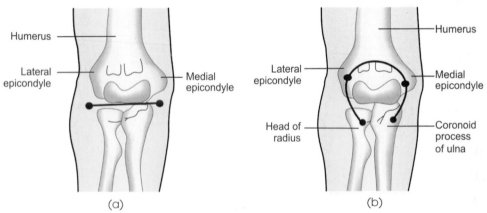

Figs 1.4a and b: Elbow joint (front)

On the back the *plane of the elbow joint* can be represented as follows (Fig. 1.5a).
- Put a point in the depression between the head of the radius and the lateral epicondyle.
- Mark the tubercle on the medial border of the coronoid process.

Join these points by a line which also represents the distal limit of the joint cavity.

The proximal limit of the joint cavity can be represented on the back of the elbow as follows (Fig. 1.5b).
- Mark a point in the depression between the head of the radius and the lateral epicondyle.
- Put a point on the tubercle, on the medial border of the coronoid process.

Draw a line from the first to the second point by an arch a little wide of the outline of the olecranon process.

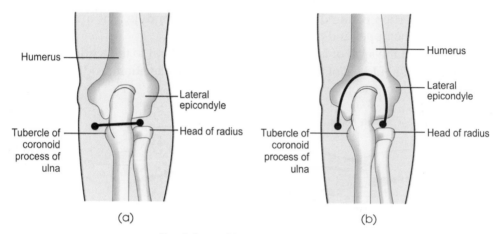

Figs 1.5a and b: Elbow joint (back)

Shoulder Joint

The joint line can be represented *on the front* as follows (Fig. 1.9):
- Put a point on the coracoid process.
  Draw a line downwards from the above point.
- The joint line can be represented *on the back* as follows (Fig. 1.7):
- Put a point on the acromial angle.
  Draw a line downwards from the above located point.

NERVES

Axillary Nerve (Fig. 1.7)

- Mark the mid point of the line joining the tip of acromion to the deltoid tuberosity.
- Put a point 2 cm above the mid point of the above line. Draw a transverse line from the second point across the deltoid muscle.

Median Nerve (Fig. 1.6)

- Draw the brachial artery (page 11)

The nerve is marked lateral to the artery in upper half and medial to it in the lower half crossing the front of the vessel in the middle.

Musculocutaneous Nerve (Fig. 1.6)

- Put a point 5 cm below the coracoid process.
- Mark the mid-point of the elevation caused by the biceps.
- Put a point lateral to the tendon of biceps.
- Join these points to get its surface marking.

Radial Nerve (Figs 1.6 and 1.7)

- Mark the commencement of the brachial artery.
- Join the insertion of the deltoid to the lateral epicondyle. Put a mark on the junction of the upper and middle-third of this line.
- Put a mark at the level of lateral epicondyle 1 cm lateral to the tendon of biceps.

    These points should be joined by a line crossing the elevation produced by long and lateral heads of triceps.

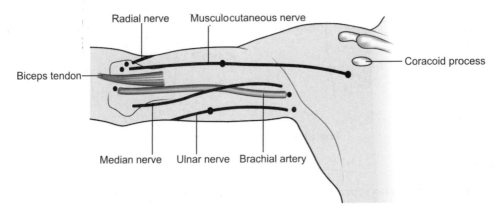

Fig. 1.6: Nerves in the front of arm

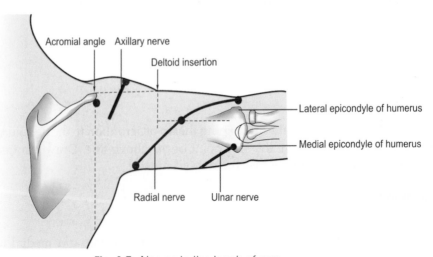

Fig. 1.7: Nerves in the back of arm

Ulnar Nerve (Fig. 1.6)

- Put a point at the commencement of the brachial artery by feeling its pulsation.
- Mark the mid-point of the brachial artery.
- Put a mark on the ulnar nerve on the back of the medial epicondyle by rolling it.

Draw a line following the medial side of the brachial artery half-way down its course. The line should then diverge to join the point on the back of medial epicondyle.

VESSELS

ARTERIES

Axillary Artery (Fig. 1.3)

Abduct the arm to a right angle.
- Mark the mid-point of clavicle.
- Put a point on the pulsation of the lower part of the axillary artery at the junction of the anterior and middle thirds of the outer axillary wall at the outlet of that space and just in front of the posterior axillary fold which becomes prominent when the abducted arm is adducted against resistance. Join these points by a broad line.

Brachial Artery (Fig. 1.8)

- Put a point on the pulsation of the lower part of axillary artery on the medial side of the arm, just in front of the posterior axillary fold.
- Mark a point at the level of the neck of the radius in the middle line of the limb. Join these points to get the surface marking.

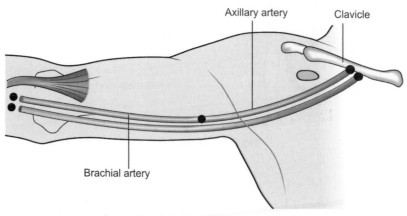

Fig. 1.8: Brachial artery

VEINS

Axillary Vein (Fig. 1.8)

- Draw like axillary artery but a little medially.

Basilic Vein (Fig. 1.9)

- Put a point on the inner side of the arm half a way between the axilla and the medial condyle.
- Mark a point on the anterior surface of the forearm below the elbow towards the medial side.

  Join the above two points by a line.

Cephalic Vein (Fig. 1.9)

- Put a point in the delto-pectoral groove below the coracoid process.
- Mark a point in front of the elbow in the groove between the brachioradialis and the biceps.

  Join these points by a line which first ascends up and then arches towards the first point.

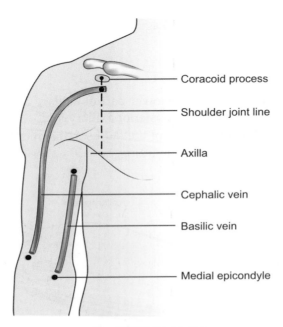

Fig. 1.9: Veins of arm

FOREARM

SURFACE LANDMARKS (Figs 1.10 and 1.11)

- **Hamate hook** can be felt distal to pisiform and nearer the centre of palm by deep pressure.
- **Pisiform bone** forms an elevation on the medial part of the base of the hypothenar eminence, and can be distinguished by tracing downwards the tendon of flexor carpi ulnaris.
- **Radius, dorsal tubercle** is situated near the middle of the posterior aspect of the lower end of the radius in line with the cleft between the index and middle fingers.
- **Radius, lower end** causes a little elevation on the lateral side of the wrist, about 1cm above the base of the thenar eminence. On the front just external to where the flexor carpi radialis tendon cuts across the two transverse creases at the wrist, there is a depression in the floor of which the lower end of radius and the tubercle of scaphoid can be felt.

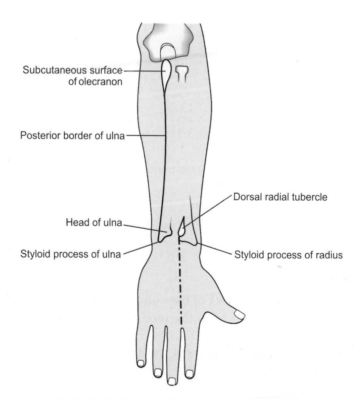

Fig. 1.10: Surface landmarks—back of forearm

- **Radius, styloid process** can be found by tracing the lateral aspect of the lower end of radius downwards. It lies 1.75 cm below and slightly on a more anterior plane than the styloid process of ulna.
- **Ulna, head** forms a round elevation on the medial side of the posterior aspect of the wrist in a pronated hand.
- **Ulna, posterior border** lies in the furrow on the back of a fully flexed forearm. It extends from the subcutaneous surface of the olecranon to the styloid process of ulna below.
- **Ulna, styloid process** can be determined by following the posterior border of ulna downwards. It will be found projecting downwards from the ulnar head.
- **Scaphoid, tubercle** is situated in the base of the thenar eminence and is partly hidden by the tendon of the flexor carpi radialis muscle. It is felt below the lower end of radius as described above.
- **Trapezium, crest** can only be recognised by applying deep pressure over the thenar muscles below and external to the tubercle of scaphoid.

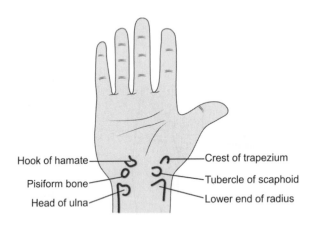

Hook of hamate
Pisiform bone
Head of ulna
Crest of trapezium
Tubercle of scaphoid
Lower end of radius

Fig. 1.11: Surface landmarks—wrist and palm

SURFACE MARKINGS

Nerves

Median Nerve (Fig. 1.12a)

- Put a point at the level of the neck of the radius in the middle line of the forearm.
- Mark a point at the wrist 1 cm to the medial side of the flexor carpi radialis tendon.

Join the above two points. At the wrist the nerve projects laterally from under cover of the palmaris longus tendon.

Posterior Interosseous Nerve (Figs 1.12a and b)

- Put a mark 1 cm lateral to the tendon of biceps at the level of lateral epicondyle of the humerus.
- Put a mark on the junction of upper and middle-third of a line joining the middle of the posterior aspect of the head of the radius to the dorsal radial tubercle of Lister.
- Mark the dorsal radial tubercle of Lister.

Join these points by a line which in the upperpart will cross the elevation produced by brachioradialis and superficial extensors.

Radial Nerve (Figs 1.12a and b)

- Put a point 1 cm lateral to the tendon of biceps at the level of lateral epicondyle of humerus.
- Mark a point at the junction of middle and lower one-third of lateral border of foream.
- Mark a point in the 'anatomical snuff box'.

Join these points.

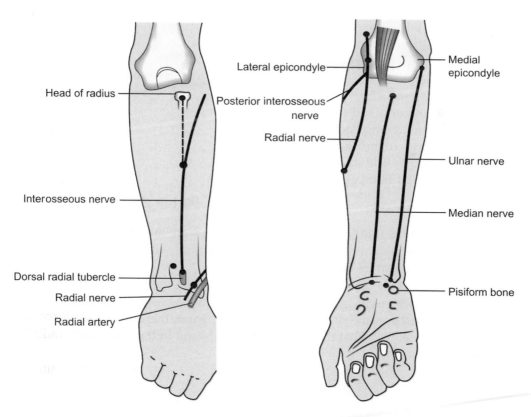

Fig. 1.12a: Nerves in back of forearm   **Fig. 1.12b:** Nerves in front of forearm

Ulnar Nerve (Fig. 1.12b)

- Put a mark on the base of the medial epicondyle of humerus.
- Mark a point at the lateral edge of the pisiform bone.

Join these two points by a line which should follow the lateral side of the tendon of flexor carpi ulnaris in the lower part of the forearm.

VESSELS

Arteries

Radial Artery (Figs 1.13 and 1.12a)

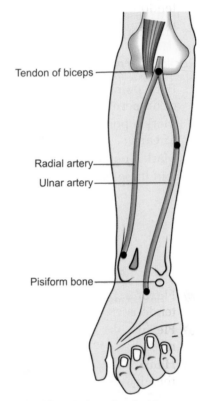

- Mark a point opposite the neck of radius on the medial side of the tendon of biceps.
- Put a mark on the pulsation of radial artery at the wrist in the interval between the tendon of flexor carpi radialis medially and the prominent lower part of the anterior border of the radius laterally.
- Put a mark on its pulsation in the 'anatomical snuff box'.

Join the first two points by a line running downwards across the medial part of the brachioradialis, and superficial extensor's elevation. The second and third points are joined by a line passing backwards across to the tendons forming the anterior boundary of 'anatomical snuff box' towards the base of the first interosseous space.

Fig. 1.13: Arteries—front of forearm

Ulnar Artery (Fig. 1.13)

- Put a point in the middle line of the forearm opposite the neck of the radius.
- Mark another point at the junction of the upper third with the lower two-thirds of the forearm near its medial border.
- Mark a point at the lateral edge of pisiform.

Join the first two points by a line which passes downwards and medially, across the elevation caused by the superficial flexors of forearm, then join the second point with the third one. Note that the ulnar artery lies lateral to the ulnar nerve.

HAND AND WRISTS

SURFACE LANDMARKS (Figs 1.14 to 1.17)

● "**Anatomical snuff box**" is an intertendinous depression seen on the lateral aspect of the wrist when the thumb is extended. Its anterior boundary is formed by the tendons of the abductor pollicis longus and the extensor pollicis brevis and the posterior one by the tendon of the extensor pollicis longus.

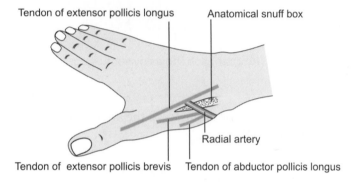

Fig. 1.14: Anatomical snuff box

● **Flexor carpiradialis** tendon. Flex the wrist against resistance. Out of the two tendons which stand out the lateral one is that of flexor carpiradialis.
● **Flexor carpiulnaris** tendon. Flex the wirst against resistance. This tendon is the medial most and will be directed towards the pisiform.
● **Hamate hook** lies 2.5 cm below and external to the pisiform bone in line with the ulnar border of the ring finger.

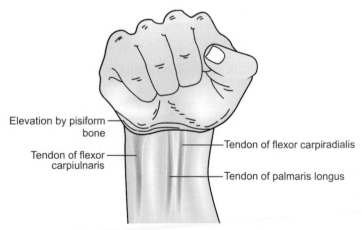

Fig. 1.15: Surface landmarks at wrist

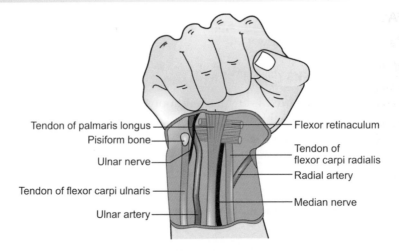

Fig. 1.16: Dissection showing structures at wrist

● **Metacarpal heads** form the prominence of the knuckles, that of the middle finger being the most prominent.

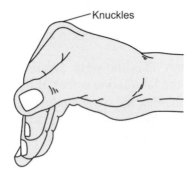

Fig. 1.17: Metacarpal heads forming the prominence of the knuckles

● **Metacarpo-phalangeal joints** are situated 2 cm distal to the creases at the junction of digits with the palm.
● **Palmaris longus tendon.** Flex the wrist against resistance. Of the two tendons which become prominent medial one is that of palmaris longus.
● **Pisiform bone** forms an elevation on the medial part of the base of the hypothenar eminence, and can be distinguished by tracing downwards the tendon of flexor carpi ulnaris.

SURFACE MARKINGS

Joints

Wrist Joint

The plane of the joint on the front (Fig. 1.18).
• Draw a line across the limb 2.5 cm proximal to the ball of the thumb.
The plane of the joint on the back (Fig. 1.19)
• Put a point a little distal to the level of the head of the ulna.

Draw a transverse line from the above point. This will be a little lower than the one drawn on the front.

Joint Cavity

• Mark the radial styloid process.
• Mark the ulnar styloid process.

Draw a curved line on the front and on the back a little higher than the lines representing the plane of the joint because the articular surface of the carpus is markedly convex from side and slightly so from before backwards.

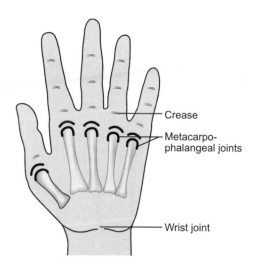

Fig. 1.18: Wrist and metacarpo-phalangeal joints

RETINACULA (Figs 1.19 and 1.20)

Extensor Retinaculum (Fig. 1.19)

- Draw a line marking the salient lower end of the anterior border of the radius above the styloid process.
- Draw a line marking the tip of styloid process of ulna and medial side of carpus.

Join these lines by a 2 cm broad oblique band on the lateral and posterior aspects of the wrist, higher on the lateral than on the medial side.

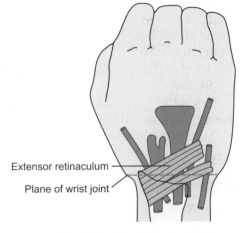

Extensor retinaculum
Plane of wrist joint

Fig. 1.19: Extensor retinaculum

Flexor Retinaculum (Fig. 1.20)

- Mark the hook of hamate.
- Mark the crest of trapezium.
- Put a point on the pisiform bone.
- Put a mark on the tubercle of scaphoid.

Join the first two points by a line concave downwards and last two points by a line concave upwards. The upper limit corresponds to the lower of the two transverse creases in front of the wrist whilst the lower limit of the ligament lies about 2 cm below.

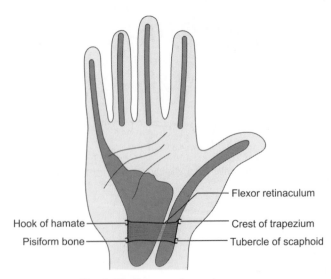

Flexor retinaculum
Hook of hamate
Pisiform bone
Crest of trapezium
Tubercle of scaphoid

Fig. 1.20: Flexor retinaculum

SYNOVIAL SHEATHS (Fig. 1.20)

Synovial sheath, common, of the flexor tendons of the digits
- Draw the flexor retinaculum.
- Mark the lateral edge of the tendon of flexor carpi ulnaris.
- Mark the medial edge of the tendon of flexor carpi radialis.

Join these lines by a line 2.5 cm above the flexor retinaculum. Narrow the sheath as it passes in the region of flexor retinaculum. Continue its medial portion distally along the lateral margin of the hypothenar eminence on the tendon of the little finger, but with this exception, the common synovial sheath does not extend beyond the level of the palmar surface of the extended thumb.

Synovial sheath, digital, of the index, middle and ring fingers
Extend in each case from the base of the distal phalanx to the head of the corresponding metacarpal bone.

VESSELS

Arteries

Deep Palmar Arch (Fig. 1.21)
- Draw the superficial arch (see below).
- Put a point just distal to the hook of hamate. Deep arch can be represented by a horizontal line 4 cm long drawn from the second point about one finger's breadth above the level of the superficial palmar arch.

Superficial Palmar Arch (Fig. 1.21)
- Put a mark on the lateral side of the pisiform bone.
- Mark the hook of hamate.
- Put a point on the centre of the palm at the level of the distal border of the extended thumb.

Draw a line starting at the first point going downwards on the medial side of the second point and then curving laterally towards the third point to form a convexity across the palm just above the upper transverse crease. It ends on the thenar eminence.

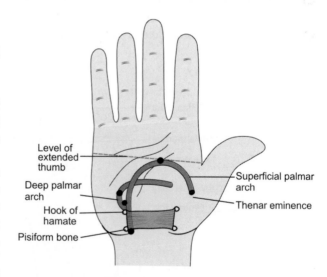

Fig. 1.21: Palmar arches

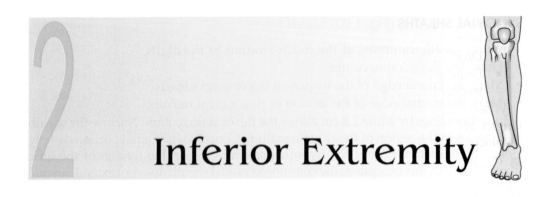

Inferior Extremity

THIGH AND GLUTEAL REGION

SURFACE LANDMARKS (Figs 2.1 and 2.2)

- **Adductor tubercle** is located by placing the flat of the hand on the medial side of thigh just above the medial condyle of femur and then slipping the hand downwards. The middle finger will come in contact with the adductor tubercle and on deep pressure the cord like tendon of adductor magnus will be recognisable immediately above the tubercle.
- **Anterior superior iliac spine** can be palpated at the lateral end of the fold of groin and is often visible.
- **Bryant's triangle** can be drawn as below.

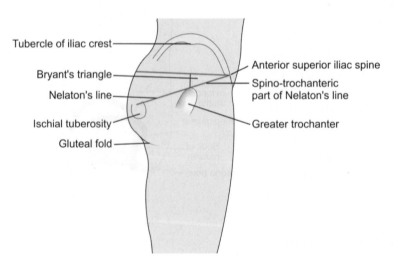

Fig. 2.1: Surface landmarks—gluteal region

- Join the two anterior superior iliac spines through the back with the subject in the recumbent posture.
- Drop a perpendicular from this line to the top of the greater trochanter.
- Draw a line from the anterior superior iliac spine to the top of the greater trochanter.

When the trochanter is displaced upward the perpendicular line is diminished in length as compared with the sound side and when it undergoes a backward displacement the spino-tronchanteric line is relatively increased in length.

⬤ **Greater trochanter of the femur** lies a hand's breadth below the tubercle of the iliac crest.

⬤ **Iliac crest** is described in section on abdomen (page 49)

   Inguinal ligament is in the fold of the groin which marks the junction of the anterior abdominal wall with the front of the thigh.

⬤ **Mid-inguinal point** is the midpoint between the anterior superior iliac spine and the symphysis pubis.

⬤ **Midpoint of the inguinal ligament** is the midpoint between the anterior superior iliac spine and the pubic tubercle.

⬤ **Nelaton's line** is a line joining the anterior superior iliac spine to the most prominent point of ischial tuberosity. It crosses the apex of the greater trochanter and the centre of the acetabulum. The extent of displacement in dislocation or in fracture of neck of femur is marked by the projection of the trochanter behind and above this line.

⬤ **Tuberosity of ischium** can be palpated 5 cm above the gluteal fold and about the same distance from the median plane.

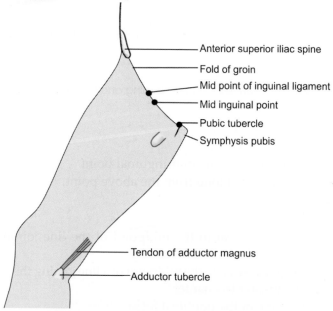

Fig. 2.2: Surface landmarks—front of thigh

SURFACE MARKING

Joint

Hip Joint (Fig. 2.3)

- Put a point 1.2 cm below the junction of lateral with the middle-third of the inguinal ligament.
- Mark another point 1.2 cm below the junction of the medial with the middle-third of the inguinal ligament.

  Join these two points to represent the joint line.

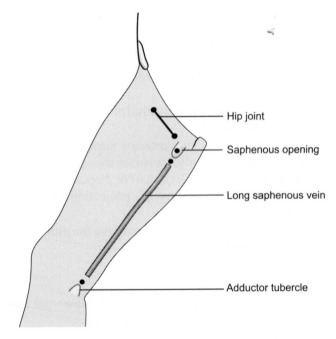

Fig. 2.3: Hip joint, saphenous opening and long saphenous vein

Nerves

Femoral Nerve (Fig. 2.4)

- Put a point 1.2 cm lateral to the mid-inguinal point
  Draw a vertical line 2.5 cm long from the above point.

Sciatic Nerve (Fig. 2.5)

- Mark a point 2.5 cm lateral to the midpoint of the line joining the posterior superior iliac spine to the ischial tuberosity.
- Put another point just medial to the midpoint of a line joining the ischial tuberosity to the apex of the greater trochanter.
- Mark the upper angle of the popliteal fossa.
  Draw a broad line passing downwards and laterally through these points.

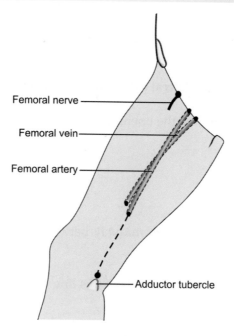

Femoral nerve

Femoral vein

Femoral artery

Adductor tubercle

Fig. 2.4: Femoral nerve and vessels

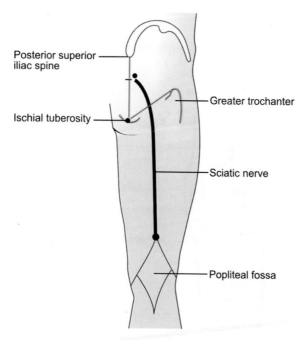

Posterior superior iliac spine

Greater trochanter

Ischial tuberosity

Sciatic nerve

Popliteal fossa

Fig. 2.5: Sciatic nerve

OPENING

Saphenous Opening (Fig. 2.3)

- Mark the pubic tubercle.
- Put a point 4 cm below and lateral to the pubic tubercle to represent the centre of the opening.
  Draw a small circle to outline the opening.

VESSELS

Arteries

Femoral Artery (Fig. 2.4)

- Take a point on the fold of groin midway between the anterior superior iliac spine and the pubic symphysis.
- Mark the adductor tubercle.
  Join these points. The upper two-thirds of this line represents the artery.

Inferior Gluteal Artery (Fig. 2.6)

- Put a point 2.5 cm lateral to the midpoint of the line joining the ischial tuberosity to the posterior superior iliac spine indicating the point of entry of the sciatic nerve into the gluteal region.
- Place a point medial to the above point. Draw a line downwards indicating the stem of the artery.

Superior Gluteal Artery (Fig. 2.6)

- Draw a line joining the posterior superior iliac spine to the apex of the greater trochanter.

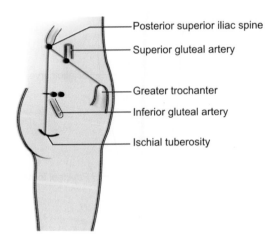

Fig. 2.6: Gluteal arteries

• Mark a point at the junction of the upper and middle-third of the above line. Draw a line upwards from the above point to indicate the stem of the artery.

VEINS

Femoral Vein (Fig. 2.4)

• Draw the femoral artery (page 26)
  The vein can be drawn close to its medial side in the upper part but behind it in most of its course and to its lateral side below.

Long Saphenous Vein (Fig. 2.3)

• Put a point a little below the centre of the saphenous opening (page 26)
• Mark the adductor tubercle.
  Join the two points by a line to represent the vein.

 LEG

SURFACE LANDMARKS (Fig. 2.7)

● **Anterior border of tibia** is distinct in most of its extent except in its lower part.
● **Head of the fibula** forms a slight elevation on the upper part of the postero-lateral aspect of the leg lying vertically below the posterior part of the lateral condyle of the femur. The common peroneal nerve can be rolled against it.
● **Lateral femoral condyle** the whole of its lateral surface can be felt through the skin. The most prominent point on its lateral aspect is termed the lateral epicondyle.
● **Lateral malleolus** forms a conspicuous projection on the lateral side of the ankle. It descends to a lower level than the medial malleolus and is placed on a more posterior plane.
● **Medial femoral condyle** has a bulging convex medial aspect which can be palpated without difficulty. The most prominent point on the medial surface of the condyle is below and a little in front of the adductor tubercle and is termed the medial epicondyle.
● **Medial malleolus,** the medial surface of the tibia is continous below with the visible prominence of medial malleolus.
● **Medial surface of tibia** is subcutaneous and easily felt.
● **Neck of fibula** is the constricted upper end of the shaft of fibula immediately below the head.
● **Popliteal fossa,** flex the knee against resistance, the fossa is the deep depression at the back of the knee.
● **Tibial condyles** form visible and palpable landmarks at the sides of ligamentum patellae. Lateral condyle is more prominent.

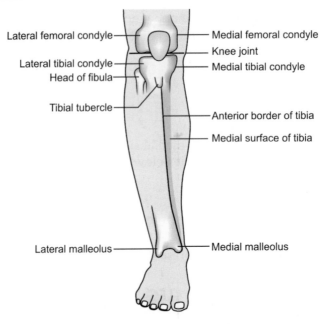

Fig. 2.7: Surface landmarks—leg

● **Tibial tubercle** is subcutaneous in its lower part only, its upper part receives the attachment of ligamentum patellae.

SURFACE MARKINGS

Joint

Knee (Fig. 2.7)

Line of the knee joint is represented by a line drawn round the limb at the level of upper margins of the tibial condyles.

Nerves

Common Peroneal Nerve (Fig. 2.9)

- Mark the upper angle of the popliteal fossa.
- Mark a point on the back of the head of the fibula.
- Mark the neck of the fibula.

Draw a line from the first point along the medial side of the tendon of the biceps femoris to the second point and then curve it downwards and forwards round the neck of the fibula.

Deep Peroneal Nerve (Fig. 2.8)

- Put a point on the lateral aspect of the neck of fibula.

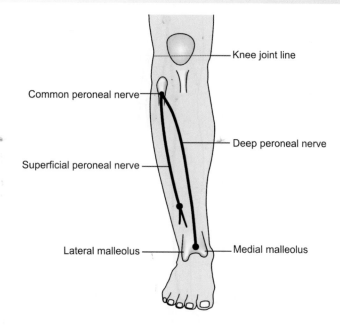

Fig. 2.8: Peroneal nerves

- Mark a point midway between the two malleoli.
  Draw a line through these points directed downwards and medially

Superficial Peroneal Nerve (Fig. 2.8)
- Mark the lateral aspect of the neck of the fibula.
- Put the peroneus longus into contraction by everting and plantar flexing the foot.
- Mark a point on its anterior border, at the junction of the middle and lower-third of leg to indicate the place where the nerve pierces the deep fascia.
  Draw a line joining these points and divide it into lateral and medial branches which gradually diverge as they descend to reach the dorsum of the foot.

Tibial Nerve (Fig. 2.9)
- Put a point on the upper limit of the popliteal fossa.
- Put another point on the lower limit of the popliteal fossa.
- Mark a point midway between the medial malleolus and the tendocalcaneus. Join these points by a line.

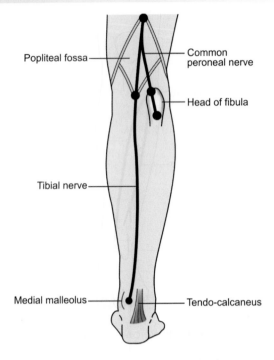

Fig. 2.9: Common peroneal and tibial nerves

VESSELS

Arteries

Anterior Tibial Artery (Fig. 2.10)

- Mark a point 2.5 cm below the medial side of the head of the fibula.
- Put a mark midway between the two malleoli.
  Draw a line joining these points and running downwards and slightly medially.

Popliteal Artery (Fig. 2.11)

- Draw a horizontal line on the back of the thigh at the junction of the middle and lower-third of the thigh.
- Draw a line to represent the level of the knee joint.
- Draw the middle line of the back of the limb between the above two horizontal lines.
- Put a point 2.5 cm medial to the middle line of the back of the limb on the first horizontal line.
- Put a mark on the back at the level of the tibial tubercle.
  Join the first point to the meeting place of the second horizontal line with the midline of the back of the thigh and extend this line to the third point.

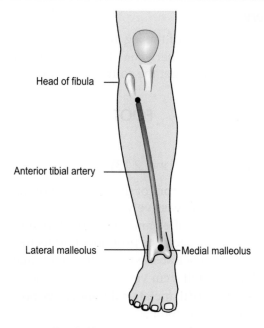

Head of fibula

Anterior tibial artery

Lateral malleolus — Medial malleolus

Fig. 2.10: Anterior tibial artery

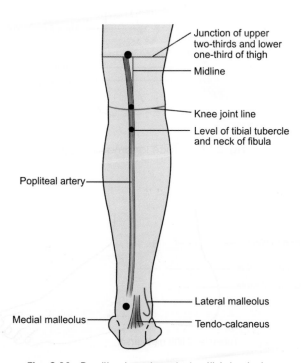

Junction of upper
two-thirds and lower
one-third of thigh

Midline

Knee joint line

Level of tibial tubercle
and neck of fibula

Popliteal artery

Lateral malleolus

Medial malleolus — Tendo-calcaneus

Fig. 2.11: Popliteal and posterior tibial arteries

Posterior Tibial Artery (Fig. 2.11)

- Put a point in the middle line of the leg at the level of the neck of fibula.
- Mark another point midway between the medial malleolus and the tendo-calcaneus. Join these points to get the course of the artery.

 # FOOT

SURFACE LANDMARKS (Figs 2.12 and 2.13)

- **Head of the talus,** lies 3 cm in front of the lower end of the tibia and can both be seen and felt when the foot is passively inverted.
- **Medial cuneiform bone,** dorsiflex and invert the foot and follow the tendon of tibialis anterior, which thus becomes prominent, to its insertion into this bone.
- **Peroneal tubercle** lies 2 cm below the tip of the lateral malleolus.
- **Sustentaculum tali** can be felt 2 cm vertically below the medial malleolus.
- **Tubercle on the base of the fifth metatarsal bone** can be both seen and felt halfway along the lateral border of the foot.
- **Tuberosity of the navicular bone** is a very conspicuous bony landmark and can be felt 2.5 cm in front of the sustentaculum tali.

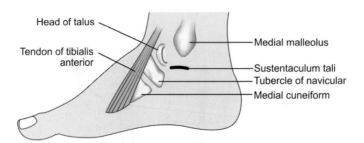

Fig. 2.12: Surface landmarks—foot

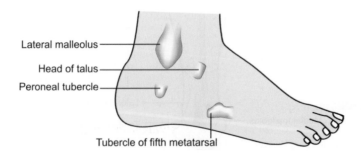

Fig. 2.13: Surface landmarks—foot

SURFACE MARKINGS

Joints

Metatarsophalangeal Joint Line (Fig. 2.15)

• Draw this line 2.5 cm behind the webs of the toes.

Mid-tarsal joint (calcaneocuboid and talonavicular) (Fig. 2.15)

• Put a point 2 cm behind the tubercle on the base of the fifth metatarsal bone.
• Mark a point on the head of talus.
  Join these two points to indicate the joint line.

Tarso-metatarsal Joint Line (Fig. 2.15)

• Mark the tubercle of the fifth metatarsal bone.
• Put a point 2.5 cm in front of the tuberosity of the navicular to indicate the tarso-metatarsal joint of the great toe.
  Join these points to get the joint line.

Nerves and Vessels

Dorsalis Pedis Artery (Fig. 2.15)

• Put a point midway between the two malleoli.
• Mark the proximal end of the first inter-metatarsal space.
  Join these two points by a line.

Lateral Plantar Artery and Nerve (Fig. 2.14)

• Put a point midway between the medial malleolus and the prominence of the heel.
• Mark a point 2.5 cm medial to the tubercle of the fifth metatarsal bone.
• Put a third point at the proximal end of the first inter-metatarsal space.
  Connect these points by a line going forward and laterally and then medially.

Medial Plantar Artery and Nerve (Fig. 2.14)

• Put a point midway between the medial malleolus and the prominence of the heel.
• Mark a point in the first interdigital cleft at the level of the navicular bone.
  Draw a line joining these points.

Retinacula

Flexor Retinaculum (Fig. 2.14)

• Draw a 2.5 cm broad band passing downwards and backwards from the medial malleolus to the medial aspect of the heel.

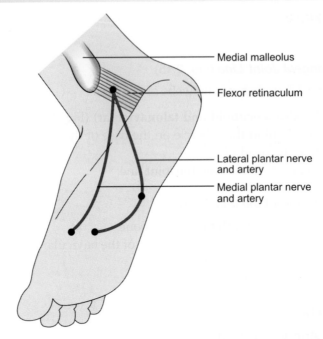

Fig. 2.14: Plantar nerves and vessels

- Medial malleolus
- Flexor retinaculum
- Lateral plantar nerve and artery
- Medial plantar nerve and artery

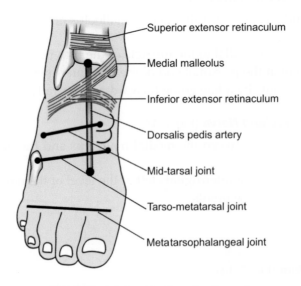

Fig. 2.15: Joints of foot and retinacula

- Superior extensor retinaculum
- Medial malleolus
- Inferior extensor retinaculum
- Dorsalis pedis artery
- Mid-tarsal joint
- Tarso-metatarsal joint
- Metatarsophalangeal joint

Its lower border runs from the tip of the malleolus to the medial tubercle of the calcaneum.

Inferior Extensor Retinaculum (Fig. 2.15)

- Draw a band 1.5 cm wide passing medially on the dorsum of the foot

On the medial side of the tendons of the extensor digitorum longus, the band divides into two diverging limbs, each 1 cm wide. The upper limb passes to the medial malleolus, the lower passes round the medial aspect of the foot to gain the plantar aspect.

Superior Extensor Retinaculum

- Draw a 3 cm wide band from the anterior border of the triangular subcutaneous area of fibula to the lower part of the anterior borders of the tibia.

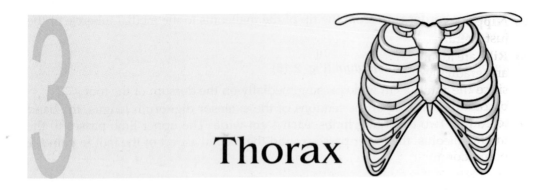

Thorax

SURFACE LANDMARKS (Figs 3.1 and 3.2)

- **Apex beat of heart** can be located by first putting the whole palm of the hand in contact with the chest wall and asking the person to bend a little forwards. When pulsation is detected its exact position is best determined with the pulp of the fingers. The apex beat is taken as the lowermost and outermost point at which the finger is distinctly forced up with each beat of the heart. It lies in health in the 5th space about 1.25 cm inside the mid-clavicular line or roughly a little medial to the left nipple.
- **Infra-sternal angle** or subcostal angle is formed at the meeting place of the two subcostal margins.

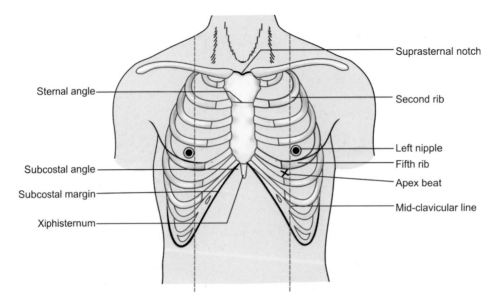

Fig. 3.1: Surface landmarks—thorax

● **Nipple** is more constant in position in men; it lies in the fourth intercostal space just lateral to the mid-clavicular line.

● **Ribs** are identified by first locating the second rib and then passing downwards and gradually going further from the sternum. This is desirable to avoid confusion since the interval between the cartilages of the fifth, sixth and seventh ribs becomes narrower as they approach the sternum. In practice, it is usually simpler to count interspaces then ribs. The first rib is difficult to palpate, but the first interspace can be located just below the clavicle and can be used as a starting point. Counting of ribs from the 12th rib upwards is unreliable. The 12th rib may be absent or it may be too short to project lateral to the erector spinae muscle. Apart from this in 1.2% of the subjects a lumbar "Gorilla" rib may be associated with the fifth lumbar vertebra.

● **Sternal angle (angle of Louis)** is usually palpable and is sometimes visible about 5 cm below the suprasternal notch of the manubrium sterni. It serves as a reference point in counting the ribs. Each second costal cartilage extends laterally from the angle.

● **Subcostal margin** can be clearly seen and is formed by the costal cartilages of 7th, 8th, 9th and 10th ribs.

● **Suprasternal notch** is visible at the upper border of manubrium between the sternal heads of sternomastoid muscles.

● **Thoracic spine third** lies opposite the medial end of the spine of the scapula.

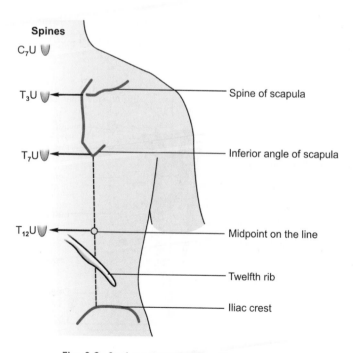

Fig. 3.2: Surface landmarks—thorax

- **Thoracic spine seventh,** lies opposite the inferior angle of scapula when the arm is in adduction.
- **Thoracic spine twelfth,** lies opposite the mid-point of a line drawn from the inferior angle of scapula to the iliac crest.
- **Xiphisternal joint** may be felt as a transverse ridge at the apex of the infra-sternal angle.
- **Xiphisternum** lies in the depression of infra-sternal angle.

SURFACE MARKINGS

Vessels

Arteries

Aorta (Fig. 3.3)
  i. **Ascending aorta**
      - Draw two parallel lines 2.5 cm apart starting from the medial end of the left third intercostal space and going upwards and to the right as far as the right half of the sternal angle.
  ii. **Arch of aorta**
      - Mark the right extremity of the sternal angle.
      - Put a point on the centre of manubrium.
      - Mark the sternal extremity of the left second costal cartilage.
        Draw a line through these points to represent the outer convexity
 iii. **Descending thoracic aorta**
      - Mark the sternal end of the left second costal cartilage.
      - Draw the transpyloric plane (page 51) put a point 2 cm above it in the median line.

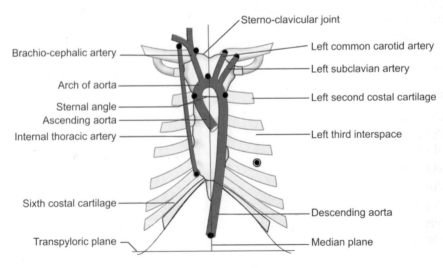

Fig. 3.3: Arteries—thorax

The aorta can be drawn out as a band 2.5 cm broad which runs downwards and medially from the first to the second point.

Brachio-cephalic Artery (Fig. 3.3)

- Mark the centre of the manubrium.
- Put a point on the right sterno-calvicular joint.
  Draw a broad line connecting these points.

Internal Thoracic Artery Right or Left (Fig. 3.3)

- Put a point 2 cm above the sternal end of the clavicle.
- Mark the sternal end of the sixth costal cartilage.
  Draw the median plane.

Join the first and second points by a line which should be 8.5 cm from the median line.

Left Common Carotid Artery (Fig. 3.3)

- Mark a point a little to the left of the centre of manubrium.
- Put a point on the left sterno-clavicular joint.
  Draw a broad line joining these points (For cervical part see page 79)

Left Subclavian Artery (Fig. 3.3)

- Put a point on the centre of the left border of manubrium sterni.
- Mark a point on the left sterno-clavicular joint.
  Draw a broad line joining these points (For cervical part see page 79)

Pulmonary Trunk (Fig. 3.4)

- Draw two parallel lines 2.5 cm apart starting and lying partly behind the left third cartilage and partly behind the sternum and ending at the 2nd left costal cartilage.

Duct

Thoracic Duct (Fig. 3.4)

- Draw the transpyloric and median planes.
- Put a point 2 cm above the transpyloric plane very slightly to the right of median plane.
- Mark the midpoint of sternal angle.
- Put a point 2 cm from the median plane and 2.5 cm above the left clavicle.
- Put another point 1.2 cm lateral to the third point.

Join these points by a line which ascends up then goes laterally through these points and then turns downwards to end behind the clavicle.

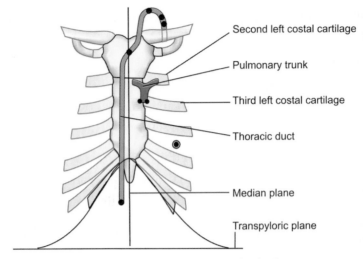

Fig. 3.4: Pulmonary trunk and thoracic duct

Veins

Left Brachiocephalic Vein (Fig. 3.5)

- Mark the sternal end of the left clavicle.
- Put a mark on the lower border of the right first costal cartilage close to the sternum.

Join these points by two parallel lines 1.5 cm apart going behind the upper half of the manubrium.

Right Brachiocephalic Vein (Fig. 3.5)

- Mark the medial end of the right clavicle.
- Put a mark on the lower border of the right first costal cartilage close to the sternum.

Join these points by two parallel lines 1.5 cm apart.

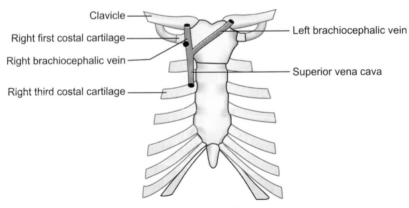

Fig. 3.5: Veins—thorax

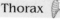

Superior Vena Cava (Fig. 3.5)

• Mark a point near the sternal end of the lower border of the right first costal cartilage.

• Put a point near the sternal end of the upper border of the right 3rd costal cartilage.

Draw a line 2 cm wide joining these points partly under cover of the right margin of the sternum.

VISCERA

Heart

Cardiac Orifices (Fig. 3.6)

Pulmonary orifice

• Draw a horizontal line 2.5 cm long partly behind the upper border of the left third costal cartilage and partly behind the sternum.

Aortic orifice

• Draw a line 3 cm long downwards and to the right from the medial end of the left third intercostal space.

Left atrioventricular or mitral orifice

• Draw a line 3 cm long passing downwards and to the right lying behind the left margin of the sternum opposite the left fourth costal cartilage.

Right atrioventricular or tricuspid orifice

• Draw a line 4 cm long beginning in the median plane opposite the fourth costal cartilage and passing downwards and slightly to the right.

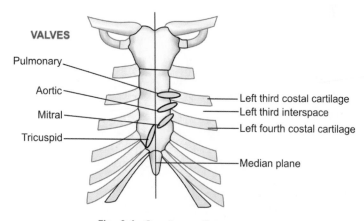

Fig. 3.6: Cardiac orifices

Sternocostal Surface (Fig. 3.7)

i. Right border
- Put a point 1.2 cm from the margin of sternum on the upper border of the right 3rd costal cartilage.
- Put a point in the right fourth interspace 3.7 cm from the median plane.
- Mark the end of the right sixth costal cartilage.
  Draw a line joining these points with a gentle convexity to the right.

ii. Lower border
- Put a point on the end of the right sixth costal cartilage.
- Mark the xiphisternal junction.
- Locate the apex beat (see page 36).
  Draw a line joining these points.

iii. Left border
- Mark the apex beat.
- Put a point 1.2 cm from the sternal margin on the lower border of the left second costal cartilage.
  Join these points by a line with an upward convexity.

iv. Upper border
  Join the upper ends of the right and left borders.

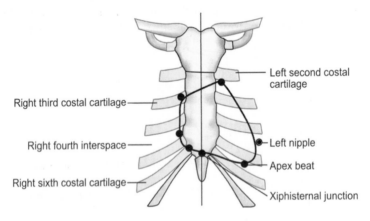

Right third costal cartilage

Right fourth interspace

Right sixth costal cartilage

Left second costal cartilage

Left nipple

Apex beat

Xiphisternal junction

Fig. 3.7: Heart sternocostal surface

Lungs (Figs 3.8 to 3.10)

Apex (Fig. 3.8)

- Put a point in the neck 2.5 cm above the medial third of the clavicle.
  Draw a convex line upwards through this point

Anterior Border (Fig. 3.8)

i. **Right lung**
- Mark the right sterno-clavicular joint.
- Put a mark on the midpoint of the sternal angle.
- Mark the sixth right chondro-sternal junction.

Join these points to represent the anterior margin of right lung.

ii. **Left lung**
- Mark the left sterno-clavicular joint.
- Put a mark on the midpoint of the sternal angle.
- Mark the fourth left chondro-sternal junction.
- Put another point on the sixth costal cartilage 2.5 cm from the left margin of the sternum.

Join these points by a line which becomes concave between the last two points to represent the cardiac notch.

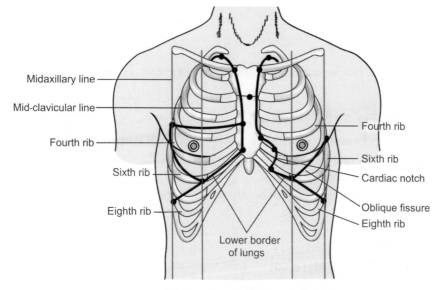

Fig. 3.8: Lungs—borders and fissures

Inferior Border (Figs 3.8 to 3.10)

- Put a mark on the sixth chondro-sternal junction for *right lung* and on the 6th costal cartilage 2.5 cm from the left margin of the sternum for *left lung*.
- Draw the mid-clavicular line and put a mark where it cuts with sixth rib.
- Draw the midaxillary line and put a mark where it cuts the eighth rib.
- Mark a point 2 cm lateral to the tenth thoracic spine.
  Join these points by a line which goes slightly upwards on the back.

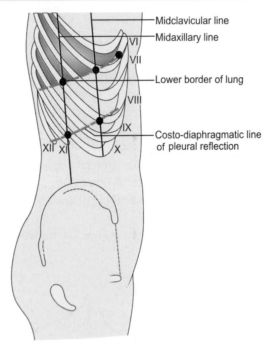

Midclavicular line
Midaxillary line
Lower border of lung
Costo-diaphragmatic line
of pleural reflection

Fig. 3.9: Lower border of lung and costo-diaphragmatic reflection of pleura

Posterior Border (Fig. 3.10)

- Put a point 2 cm from the midline at the level of spinous process of T_{10}.
- Mark a point 2 cm lateral to the second thoracic spine.
  Join these points by a vertical line.
  Apices of the lungs at the back can be drawn by a line convex upwards 5 cm from the midline.

Fissures and Lobes

Oblique Fissures (Figs 3.8 and 3.10)

- Put a point 2 cm lateral to the second thoracic spine.
- Mark a point 3 cm lateral to and at the level of the nipple.
- Put another point on the 6th costal cartilage 7.5 cm from the median plane.

The upper part of the fissure can be drawn by a line joining the first two points or following the vertebral border of the scapula when the corresponding hand of the subject has been placed on the back of the head. The second and third points can then be joined by continuing this line on the front of the chest, downwards and medially.

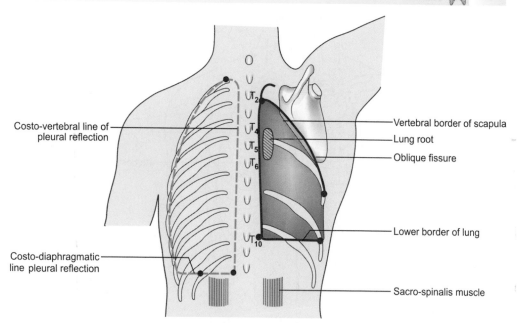

Costo-vertebral line of pleural reflection

Costo-diaphragmatic line pleural reflection

Vertebral border of scapula

Lung root

Oblique fissure

Lower border of lung

Sacro-spinalis muscle

Fig. 3.10: Lower and posterior borders of lung and respective pleural reflections

Transverse Fissure of the Right Lung (Fig. 3.8)

- Put a point in the median plane at the level of 4th costal cartilage.
- Draw the midaxillary line.

Join the first point to the mid-axillary line by a transverse line along the right fourth costal cartilage.

Roots of Lungs (Fig. 3.10)

- Mark the 4th, 5th and 6th thoracic spines.

Draw vertical lines midway between the posterior median line and vertebral border of scapula at the level of the spines marked.

Lines of Pleural Reflection

Right Costo-mediastinal Reflection (Fig. 3.11)

- Mark the sterno-clavicular joint.
- Put another mark on the mid-point of the sternal angle.
- Mark the xiphisternal joint.
  Draw a line joining these points.

Left Costo-mediastinal Reflection (Fig. 3.11)

- Mark the sterno-clavicular joint.
- Mark the mid-point of sternal angle.

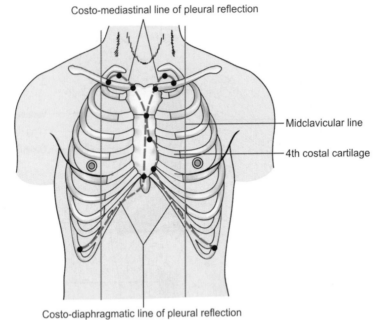

Costo-mediastinal line of pleural reflection

Midclavicular line

4th costal cartilage

Costo-diaphragmatic line of pleural reflection

Fig. 3.11: Pleural reflections

- Put another point in the midline at the level of left fourth costal cartilage.
- Mark the xiphisternal joint.

Draw a line to joint the first three points then carry it to the left to reach the sternal margin and follow that margin to reach the left extremity of xiphisternal joint.

Costo-diaphragmatic Reflection

- Mark the xiphisternal joint.
- Draw the mid-clavicular line and put a mark where it passes over the 8th rib.
- Draw the mid-axillary line and mark the point where it crosses the 10th rib.
- Mark the tip of the twelfth costal cartilage or the lateral border of the sacro-spinalis muscle.
- Put a point 2 cm lateral to the upper border of the twelfth thoracic spine.

Draw a line joining these points. On the *right side* the pleura descends below the costal margin in the right xiphocostal angle.

Cervical Pleura (Fig. 3.11)

- Mark the sterno-clavicular joint.
- Put a point on the junction of the medial and middle-third of the clavicle.
- Put another point between the above two points but 3.5 cm above the clavicle. Draw a line joining these points.

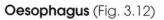

Oesophagus (Fig. 3.12)

The cervical, thoracic and abdominal parts can be marked as under
- Mark the lower border of the arch of the cricoid cartilage.
- Put a point on the median plane a little below the sternal angle.
- Mark a point on the left seventh costal cartilage 2.5 cm from the median plane.

Join these points by two parallel lines 2.5 cm apart. In connecting the first two points the lines should incline to the left in the first place, then they should curve to the right. In going to the third point they should incline to the left again.

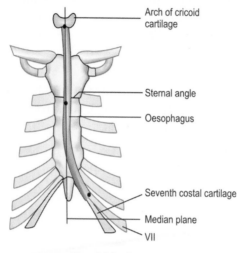

Fig. 3.12: Oesophagus

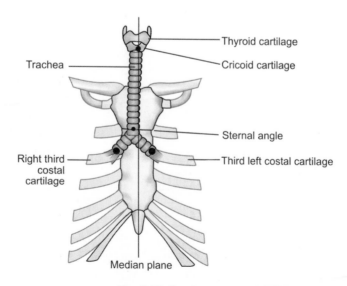

Fig. 3.13: Trachea

Trachea and Bronchi (Fig. 3.13)

Trachea (Cervical and Thoracic Parts)

- Put a point immediately below the arch of the cricoid cartilage.
- Mark a point 1 cm to the right of the centre of the sternal angle.

Draw two parallel lines 2 cm apart which should commence at the first point and incline very slightly to the right at the sternal angle.

Right Bronchus (Fig. 3.13)

- Put a point a little to the right of the centre of sternal angle.
- Mark the sternal end of the third right costal cartilage.

Draw a line 2.5 cm long joining these points.

Left Bronchus (Fig. 3.13)

- Mark a point a little to the right of the centre of the sternal angle.
- Put a point on the left third costal cartilage 3.5 cm from the median plane.

Draw a line 5 cm long joining these points.

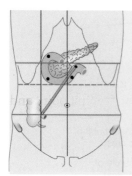

Abdomen and Pelvis

4

SURFACE LANDMARKS (Figs 4.1 and 4.2)

- **Anterior superior iliac spine** lies at the lateral end of the fold of the groin.
- **Highest point of the iliac crest** lies opposite the interval between the spines of L3 and L4.
- **Iliac crest** can be palpated throughout its whole length at the lower part of the back.
- **Linea alba** is a linear depression in the median plane.
- **Linea semilunaris** is a curved groove crossing the costal margin at or near the tip of the ninth costal cartilage and terminating below at the pubic tubercle. It corresponds to the outer border of the rectus abdominis muscle.
- **McBurney's point** (Fig. 4.3) is situated at the junction of the outer and middle-third of a line drawn from the right anterior superior iliac spine to the umbilicus. This point corresponds to the usual seat of maximum pain on palpation in an attack of appendicitis. The surface marking of the caecal orifice of the appendix does not coincide with this point.

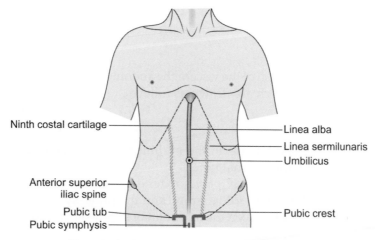

Fig. 4.1: Surface landmarks—abdomen

49

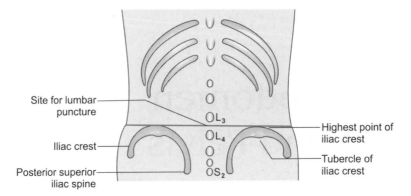

Fig. 4.2: Surface landmarks—back of abdomen

- **Posterior superior iliac spines** lie under two symmetrically placed dimples by the side of the commencement of the natal cleft.
- **Pubic crest** is the free rounded upper border of the body of the pubis and can be felt lateral to the pubic symphysis.
- **Pubic symphysis** can be felt indistinctly at the lower end of median line.
- **Pubic tubercle** is a rounded projection at the lateral extremity of the pubic crest. It is obscured by the spermatic cord which crosses its upper aspect.
- **Second sacral spine** lies on the middle of the line joining the posterior superior iliac spines.
- **Tubercle of iliac crest** lies 5 cm or more behind the anterior superior iliac spine on a level with the upper border of L5 (the transtubercular plane).
- **Umbilicus** usually lies 2.5 cm to 3.5 cm above the transtubercular plane, and corresponds to the level of the disc between L3 and L4. It is, however, very inconstant in position.

PLANES (Fig. 4.3)

For covenience of description of the viscera the abdomen is divided by certain sagittal and horizontal planes which are drawn as follows.

Sagittal Planes

i. *Median vertical plane* extends in the midline from the symphysis pubis to the middle point at supra-sternal notch.

ii. *Right and left lateral vertical planes* extend vertically up from midway between the anterior superior iliac spine and the pubic symphysis to a point on the clavicle midway between the midpoint of supra-sternal notch and acromio-clavicular joint.

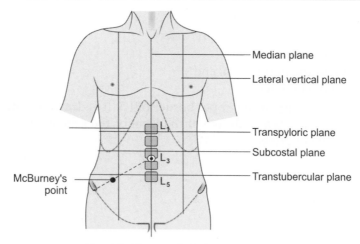

Fig. 4.3: Planes of abdomen

Transverse Planes

i. *Transpyloric plane (of Addison).* It is indicated by a line midway between the suprasternal notch and the symphysis pubis. It approximately lies midway between the umbilicus and xiphisternal joint and crosses at the tip of ninth costal cartilage. It lies at the lower border of LI.

This "key" plane of abdomen passes through (Fig. 4.4)
- pylorus,
- inferior margin of liver 2.5 cm to the right of the midline,
- neck of the gall bladder,

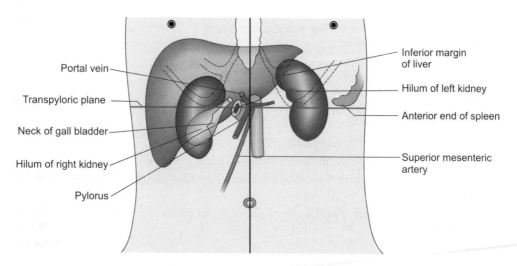

Fig. 4.4: Transpyloric plane—the 'Key' plane of abdomen

- anterior end of the spleen,
- origin of superior mesenteric artery,
- neck of pancreas,
- origin of the portal vein, and
- hili of the kidneys.

ii. *Subcostal plane* lies at the upper border of L3. It is drawn below the 10th rib.

iii. *Transtubercular plane* is drawn at the level of the tubercle on the iliac crest. It lies near the upper border of L5.

SURFACE MARKINGS

Abdominal Wall

Inguinal Canal (Fig. 4.5)

- Mark the internal abdominal ring 1.25 cm above the mid-point of the inguinal ligament.
- Put a point immediately above the pubic tubercle to mark the external ring. Join these points by two parallel lines 3.75 cm long to indicate the canal.

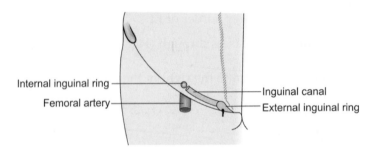

Fig. 4.5: Inguinal canal

Arteries

Abdominal Aorta (Fig. 4.6)

- Draw the median and transpyloric planes.
- Put a point on the median plane 2.5 cm above the transpyloric plane.
- Mark a point 1.2 cm below the umbilicus and the same distance from the median plane.

  Join these points by two parallel lines about 2 cm apart.

Coeliac Artery (Fig. 4.6)

- It can be represented by a small circle on the median plane 2.5 cm above the transpyloric plane.

Common Iliac Artery and External Iliac Artery (Fig. 4.6)

- Put a point 1.2 cm below the umbilicus and the same distance from the median plane (bifurcation of aorta).
- Mark the mid-point between the anterior superior iliac spine and the pubic tubercle.

Draw a broad line joining these points and presenting a slight convexity to the lateral side.

    – Upper one-third will represent common iliac artery.
    – Lower two-thirds will represent external iliac artery.

Hepatic Artery (Fig. 4.6)

- Place a point on the median plane 2.5 cm above the transpyloric plane.
- Mark a point 2.5 cm below and to the right of the first point.
- Put a point 3 cm vertically above the second point.
  Join these points by a line to get the marking of the artery.

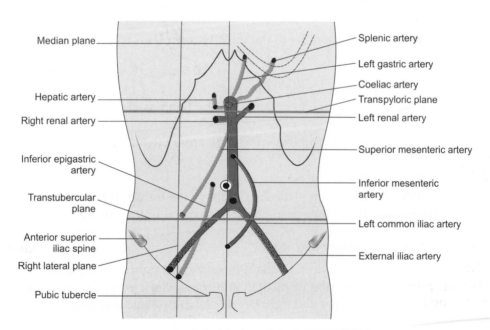

Fig. 4.6: Arteries of abdomen

Inferior Epigastric Artery (Fig. 4.6)

- Put a point midway between the anterior superior iliac spine and the pubic symphysis.
- Mask a point 1.25 to 2.5 cm outside the umbilicus.

Join these two points to indicate the course of this artery which forms the outer boundary of inguinal triangle of Hesselbach.

Inferior Mesenteric Artery (Fig. 4.6)

- Put a point 2.5 cm above the umbilicus and 1.2 cm to the left of the median plane.
- Mark another point 4 cm below the umbilicus.

Join these points by a line which runs downwards and slightly to the left from the first to the second point.

Left Gastric Artery (Fig. 4.6)

- Put a point on the median plane 2.5 cm above the transpyloric plane.
- Place a point 2.5 cm to the left of the median plane on seventh costal cartilage to represent the cardiac orifice of the stomach.

Join these points by a line going upwards and to the left.

Renal Arteries (Fig. 4.6)

i. **Right**
- Put a point in the median plane 1.5 cm below the transpyloric plane.
- Place another point 4 cm lateral to first point and below the transpyloric plane.

Draw a broad line parallel to the transpyloric plane and joining the above two points.

ii. **Left**
- Put the first point as for the right artery.
- Mark the second point 4 cm lateral to the first but above the transpyloric plane.

Join these points by a broad line which will cross the transpyloric plane.

Splenic Artery (Fig. 4.6)

- Mark a point on the median plane 2.5 cm above the transpyloric plane.

Draw a wavy line 10 cm long going to the left and slightly upwards.

Superior Mesenteric Artery (Fig. 4.6)

- Draw the median, transpyloric, trans-tubercular and right lateral planes.

Join the point of intersection of median and transpyloric planes to the point of intersection of transtubercular and right lateral planes by a line gently convex to the left.

Veins

Common and External Iliac Veins (Fig. 4.7)

- Put a point just below the trans-tubercular plane 2.5 cm to the right of the median plane indicating the commencement of the inferior vena cava.
- Mark a point 1 cm medial to the mid-point of the line joining the pubic symphysis to the anterior superior iliac spine.

  Join the two points by a line slightly convex to the lateral side. Upper one-third will represent the common iliac and lower two-thirds the external iliac vein.

Inferior Vena Cava (Fig. 4.7)

- Draw the transtubercular plane and the median plane.
- Put a point just below the transtubercular plane and 2.5 cm from the median plane to indicate the centre of the vessel.
- Mark the sternal end of the right sixth costal cartilage.

  Draw two vertical lines 2.5 cm apart joining these two points.

Portal Vein (Fig. 4.8)

- Draw the transpyloric and the median planes.
- Put a point on the transpyloric plane 1.2 cm to the right of the median plane.

  Draw a broad line 5 cm long and 1.5 cm wide from the above point going upwards and to the right.

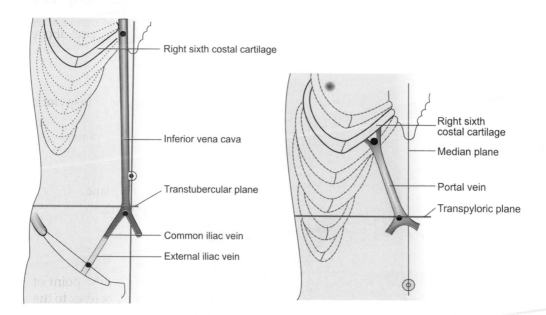

Figs 4.7 and 4.8: Veins of abdomen

Digestive System

Stomach (Fig. 4.9)

i. *Cardiac orifice*
- Draw the median plane.
- Put a mark 2.5 cm to the left of the median plane on the seventh costal cartilage.

Draw two short parallel lines 2 cm apart inclining downwards and to the left from the above point.

ii. **Pylorus**
- Draw the transpyloric plane.
- Put a point on the above plane, 1.2 cm to the right of the median plane.

Draw two short parallel lines 2 cm apart, directed upwards and to the right.

iii. **Lesser curvature**
- Join the right margin of the cardiac orifice to the upper margin of the pylorus by means of a curved J-shaped line which descends at its lowest-point below the transpyloric plane.

iv. **Fundus**
- Put a point in the left fifth intercostal space just below the nipple.

Fundus can be indicated by a line drawn from the left margin of the cardiac orfice with upward convexity reaching its summit at the above point.

v. **Greater curvature**
- Draw the subcostal plane.
- Put a point between the tips of ninth and tenth left costal cartilages.

Draw a curved line convex to the left from the fundus to the point marked and reaching downwards to the subcostal plane and then reaching the lower margin of pylorus.

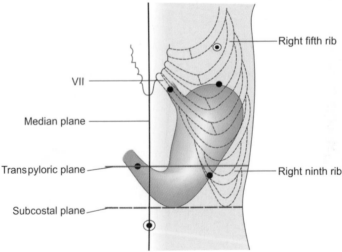

Fig. 4.9: Stomach

Small Intestine

Duodenum (Fig. 4.10)

i. **First part**
- Draw the transpyloric plane.
- Mark the pylorus of stomach by two short parallel lines 2 cm apart on the transpyloric plane 1.2 cm to the right of the median plane.
- Mark a point 2.5 cm above and to the right of the pylorus.

Join the last two points.

ii. **Second part**
- Draw the right lateral plane.
- Put a point 7.5 cm below the transpyloric plane and medial to the right lateral plane.

Draw the second part 2.5 cm wide from the end of the first part to the point described above.

iii. **Third part**
- Draw the subcostal plane.

Draw the third part transversely from the end of the second part at the level of the subcostal plane and ending just to the left of median plane.

iv. **Fourth part**
- Put a point 2.5 cm to the left of the median plane and 1 cm below the transpyloric plane to indicate the duodeno-jejunal flexure.

Join the end of the third part with this point to indicate the last part of the duodenum.

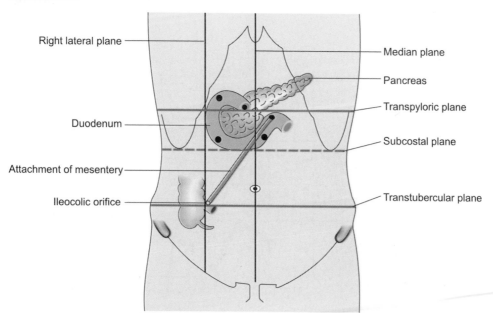

Fig. 4.10: Duodenum, mesentery and pancreas

Jejunum and Ileum

Attachment of the Mesentery of Small Intestine (Fig. 4.10)

- Draw the median, right lateral, transpyloric and trans-tubercular planes.
- Put a point 2.5 cm to the left of median plane and 1 cm below the transpyloric plane.
- Mark a point at the intersection of right lateral and trans-tubercular planes.
  Join these points to indicate the attachment of the mesentery.

Ileocolic Orifice (Fig. 4.10)

- Lies opposite the point of intersection of the transtubercular and the right lateral planes.

Large Intestine (Fig. 4.11)

   i. **Caecum**
- Draw the right lateral plane.
- Draw the trans-tubercular plane.

Mark the figure of caecum 6 cm long in the triangular area bounded by the above two planes and the fold of the groin.

      Opening of vermiform appendix
- Lies 2 cm below the junction between the right lateral and the transtubercular planes.

  ii. **Ascending colon**
- Draw the transpyloric, subcostal, transtubercular and right lateral planes.

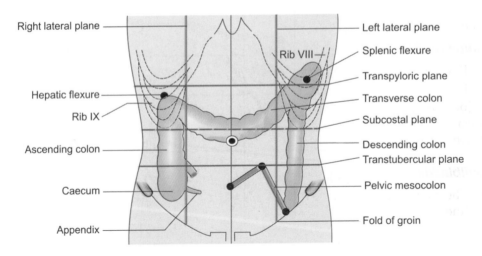

Fig. 4.11: Large intestine and pelvic mesocolon

Draw two lines 5 cm apart lying to the right of the right lateral plane starting on the transtubercular plane and ending midway between subcostal and transpyloric planes, corresponding to the upper part of ninth right costal cartilage, here the gut turns on itself to form the **hepatic flexure**.

iii. Transverse colon

- Mark a point midway between transpyloric and subcostal planes and to the right of the right lateral plane at the level of ninth costal cartilage to indicate the upper end of ascending colon.
- Put another point above the transpyloric plane to the left of the left lateral plane at the level of the left eighth costal cartilage.

Draw two lines 5 cm apart starting at the first point and descending downwards and medially to the umbilicus and then ascending upwards and laterally to the second point. At the second point it forms the **splenic flexure**.

iv. Descending colon

- Put a point above the transpyloric plane to the left of left lateral plane at the level of the left eighth costal cartilage.
- Mark another point on the fold of the groin.

Draw two lines 2 cm apart starting at the first point and ending at the second and lying wholly to the left of the lateral plane.

Attachment of Pelvic Mesocolon (Fig. 4.11)

- Put a point on the left fold of groin about midway.
- Mark a point on the trans-tubercular plane 2.5 cm medial to its junction with the left lateral plane.
- Place a third point on the midline midway between the umbilicus and pubic symphysis.

Join the first point with the second and second with the third point.

Extra-hepatic biliary Apparatus

Common Bile Duct (Fig. 4.12)

- Put a point in the sixth intercostal space 2.5 cm from the median plane.
- Draw the subcostal plane and mark a point on it 1.75 cm from the median plane.

Join these points by a line 7.5 cm 'long which should run first downwards and inwards to the costal margin, then run parallel to the midline for 4 cm and then downwards and laterally for 2 cm to the point on the subcostal plane.

Gallbladder (Fig. 4.12)

- The fundus can be marked in the angle between the right costal margin and linea semilunaris.

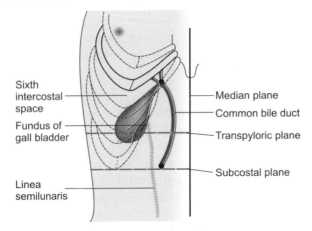

Fig. 4.12: Hepatobiliary tract

Liver (Fig. 4.13)

   i. **Upper border**
- Mark the xiphisternal joint.
- Put a point a little below the right nipple.
- Mark a point a little below and medial to the left nipple.

  Draw a line through the xiphisternal joint ascending to the right point and ascending less sharply to the left point.

  ii. **Right border**
- Put a point 1 cm just below the tip of the right tenth costal cartilage. Draw a convex line from below the right nipple to the above point.

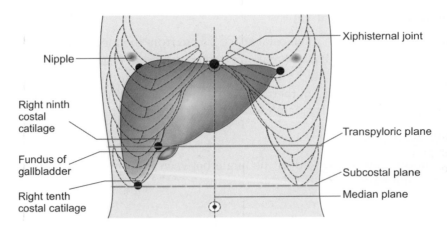

Fig. 4.13: Liver

iii. **Lower border**
- Draw the median and transpyloric planes.
- Mark the tip of the right ninth costal cartilage.

Join the lower end of the right border to the left end of the upper border by a line crossing the median plane at the transpyloric plane. This border should show a slight notch opposite the tip of the ninth right costal cartilage for the fundus of gall bladder.

Pancreas (Fig. 4.10)

i. **Head:** It can be indicated by drawing the curve of the duodenum thus:
- Draw the transpyloric, subcostal, medial and right lateral planes.
- Put a point on the transpyloric plane 1.2 cm to the right of the median plane.
- Mark a second point 2.5 cm above and to the right of the first point.
- Put a third point 7.5 cm below the transpyloric plane and medial to the right lateral plane.
- Mark a fourth point on the subcostal plane just to the left of the median plane.
- Put a fifth point 2.5 cm to the left of the median plane and 1 cm below the transpyloric plane.

Join these five points by a curve indicating the concavity of the duodenal loop which also outlines the head of the pancreas.

ii. **Neck**
- Passes upwards and to the left and is the junction of the head and the body.

iii. **Body**
- Body can be represented by two parallel lines 10 cm long and 3 cm apart going to the left from the neck.

iv. **Tail**
- Tail extends to the left as far as the hilum of spleen.

Urogenital System

Kidneys (Anterior Surface Markings) (Fig. 4.14)

- Draw the median and transpyloric planes.
- Mark the hilum 5 cm away from the median plane. That of the right kidney a little below and of the left kidney a little above the transpyloric plane. This will be just internal to the anterior extremity of the ninth costal cartilage.

Draw the shape of the kidney 8.5 cm in length and 5 cm in breadth with the upper pole 4.2 cm and lower pole 8.5 cm away from the median plane. The left kidney should be drawn a little higher than the right.

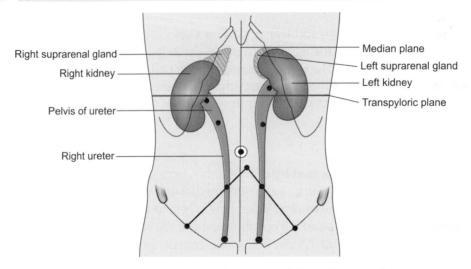

Fig. 4.14: Kidneys, ureters and supra-renals (anterior aspect)

Ureters (Anterior Surface Marking) (Fig. 4.14)

- Mark the hilum of the kidney 5 cm away from the median plane. That of the right kidney a little below and of the left kidney a little above the transpyloric plane.
- Put a point 5 cm below the transpyloric plane and same distance from the median plane.
- Mark a point at the junction of the upper and middle-third of a line drawn from a point 1.25 cm below and to the left of the umbilicus to a second point situated half way between the anterior superior iliac spine and the symphysis pubis.

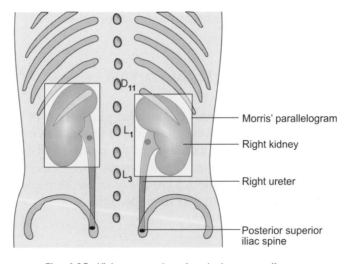

Fig. 4.15: Kidneys, ureters (posterior aspect)

- Mark the pubic tubercle.

  Draw the pelvis of the ureter between the first two points.

  Join the last two points to trace the ureter in abdomen and pelvis.

Kidneys (Posterior Surface Marking) (Fig. 4.15)

Map out the Morris' parallelogram as under
- Draw two horizontal lines through the D11 and L3 spines.
- Put two vertical lines 2.5 cm and 9.5 cm from the median plane.
- Mark the hilum of the kidney opposite the lower border of the LI spine.

  The kidneys are drawn with their long axes oblique so that the upper poles are nearer and the lower poles farther from the median plane.

Ureters (Posterior Surface Marking) (Fig. 4.15)

- Mark a point 4 cm from the median plane at the level of lower border L1.
- Locate the dimple which overlies the posterior superior iliac spine.

  Join these to get the surface marking of the ureter on the back.

Ductless Glands

Spleen (Fig. 4.16)

- Put a point 4 cm lateral to D_{10} spine to indicate the upper pole.
- Put another point on the left eleventh rib in the mid-axillary line to indicate the lower pole.

  Join these two ends by a curved line extending upwards and forwards to the ninth rib. The long axis of the spleen lies in the line of the tenth rib and width of the spleen extends throughout the ninth and tenth intercostal spaces.

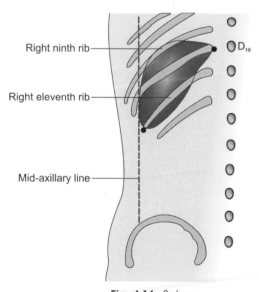

Right ninth rib

Right eleventh rib

Mid-axillary line

D_{10}

Fig. 4.16: Spleen

Suprarenals (Fig. 4.14)

Left gland
- Draw the left kidney

Draw a semilunar figure 4.5 cm long and 2 cm wide closely applied to the medial border of the left kidney above the hilum.

Right gland
- Draw the right kidney.

Draw a triangle measuring 3 cm long and 3 cm wide placed at the upper pole of the right kidney.

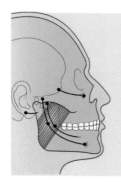

Head and Neck

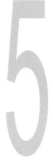

5

 FACE AND CRANIUM

SURFACE LANDMARKS (Figs 5.1 to 5.4)

● **Asterion** is placed about 2 cm behind and 1.25 cm above the superior part of the posterior border of the mastoid process.

● **Bregma** can be marked at the centre of the line drawn across the vertex from one external auditary meatus to the other, the head being in the usual erect position.

● **Condyloid process** can be felt to pass downwards and forwards immediately in front of the lower part of the tragus when the mouth is opened.

● **External occipital protuberance** can be felt at the upper end of the nuchal furrow on the back of neck.

● **Fronto-zygomatic suture** can be recognised as a slight irregular depression on the lateral orbital margin.

● **Gonion or the angle of mandible** can be seen and palpated below and in front of the lobule of the ear. It is the outer margin of the angle of mandible.

● **Inion** is the highest point on the external occipital protuberance.

● **Lambda** corresponds to an irregular depression above and in front of the maximum occipital point which is a backward convexity above the external occipital protuberance. It is situated about 7 cm above the external occipital protuberance.

● **Mastoid process** is hidden by the lobule of the ear. Its anterior border and lateral aspect can be felt easily. The insertions of sternomastoid and splenius capitis obscure its posterior border and the tip.

● **Mental protuberance**, the projection is easily identifiable at the chin.

● **Nasion** is a well marked depression at the root of the nose and overlies the junction of frontonasal and internasal sutures.

● **Pre-auricular point** is situated immediately in front of the upper part of the tragus of the ear and the pulsation of superficial temporal artery can be felt there.

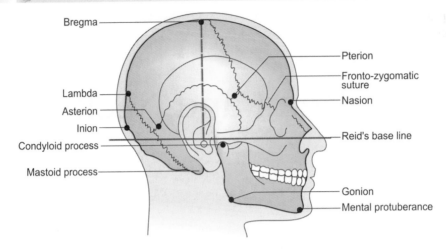

Fig. 5.1: Surface landmarks—face and cranium

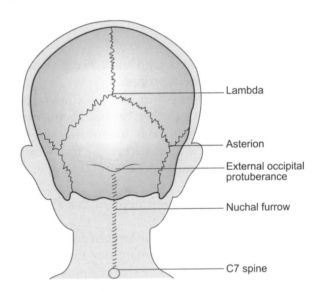

Fig. 5.2: Surface landmarks—back of Head

● **Pterion** is neither a visible nor a palpable surface landmark. Its centre can be located approximately 3.5 cm behind and 1.5 cm above the fronto-zygomatic suture. It can also be located by placing the thumb behind the frontal process of the zygomatic bone and two fingers above the zygomatic arch. The angle thus formed lies on pterion (Stiles).

● **Reid's base line** passes through a point on the lowest level of the infra-orbital margin and another point on the upper border of the external auditary meatus.

The cerebrum lies entirely above the level of this line while the cerebellum occupies the area immediately below the posterior third of this line and can be given no definite surface marking.

● **Supra-orbital notch** is present at the junction of rounded medial third and sharper lateral two-thirds of supra-orbital margin.

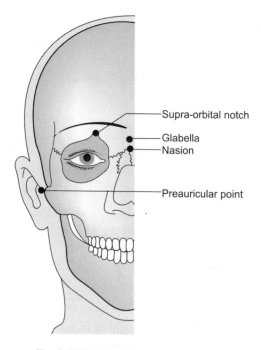

Fig. 5.3: Surface landmarks—face

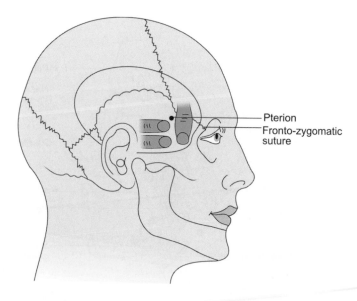

Fig. 5.4: Stile's method for locating pterion

SURFACE MARKINGS

Glands

Parotid Duct (Fig. 5.5)

- Mark the lower border of the concha of the ear.
- Put a point midway between the ala of the nose and the red margin of the upper lip.

The middle-third of the line joining these points represents the parotid duct.

Parotid Gland (Fig. 5.5)

For *anterior border* join the following points:
- Mark the upper border of the mandibular condyle.
- Take a point a little above the centre of the masseter muscle.
- Mark another point 2 cm below and behind the angle of mandible.

Upper border is drawn by a curved line below the external auditary meatus across the lobule of the ear and joining the following points:
- Upper border of the mandibular condyle.
- Mastoid process

Posterior border is a straight line joining
- The apex of mastoid process.
- A point 2 cm below and behind the angle of mandible.

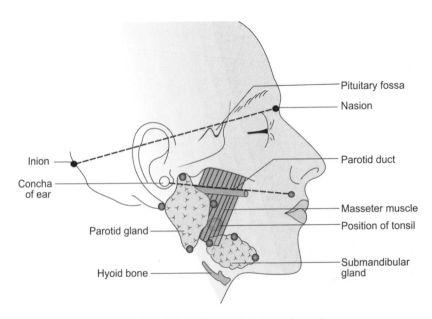

Fig. 5.5: Salivary glands and tonsil

Pituitary Fossa and Gland (Fig. 5.5)

- Lies on the straight line joining the nasion with the inion at a depth of 6–7 cm from the nasion.

Submandibular Salivary Gland (Fig. 5.5)

- Put a mark on the angle of mandible.
- Mark a point on the lower border of mandible midway between angle and the symphysis.
- Put another point midway between the above two but 1.5 cm above the lower border of mandible.
- Indicate the greater cornu of the hyoid bone by a line.
  Join these markings with an oval figure.

Tonsil (Fig. 5.5)

- Tonsil is drawn by an oval outline situated over the masseter muscle just above and in front of the angle of mandible.

Nerves

Facial Nerve (Fig. 5.6)

- Put a point on the middle of the anterior border of the mastoid process.
- Draw a horizontal line across the upper part of the lobule of the ear.
- The general transparotid course of the nerve and the direction of its buccal branch may be indicated by a line drawn forwards parallel to and below Parotid duct from the lobule of the ear (see page 68).

Lingual Nerve (Fig. 5.6)

- Put a point opposite the posterior part of the mandibular notch.
- Mark a point a little below and behind the last molar tooth.
  Draw a line downwards and forwards joining the first and second points and continue it forwards with an upward concavity along the body of the mandible.

Mandibular and Inferior Alveolar Nerves (Fig. 5.6)

- Put a point on the centre of the zygomatic arch.
- Mark the centre of the masseter muscle to represent the mandibular foramen.
- Place a point midway between upper and lower borders of the mandible and vertically below the interval between the premolar teeth to represent the mental foramen.
  Draw a line joining these points with an upward concavity. The upper vertical part of the line represents the mandibular nerve and the rest represents the inferior alveolar nerve.

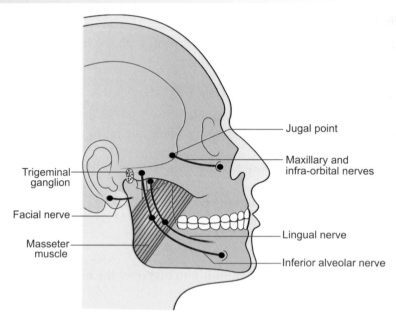

Fig. 5.6: Nerves of face

Maxillary and Infra-orbital Nerve (Fig. 5.6)

- Mark the jugal point which is the angle between the temporal border of the zygomatic bone and upper border of the zygomatic arch.
- Mark the infra-orbital foramen by a point vertically below the supra-orbital notch and 1 cm below the infra-orbital margin.

Join these two points to represent the course of the maxillary nerve and its infra-orbital branch.

Trigeminal Ganglion (Fig. 5.6)

- Lies opposite a point situated a little in front of the preauricular point. It is at a distance of 4.5–5 cm from the lateral aspect of the head.

VESSELS

Arteries

Facial Artery (Fig. 5.6)

- Mark a point at the anterior—inferior angle of the masseter muscle by palpating the artery there.
- Put a point 1.2 cm lateral to the angle of the mouth.
- Mark a point at the medial angle of the eye.

Join these points by a line which should curve forwards almost to the ala of the nose.

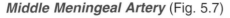

Middle Meningeal Artery (Fig. 5.7)

- Put a point a little in front of the preauricular point.
- Mark another point 2 cm above the middle of the zygomatic arch.

Join the above two points by a line which goes forward and slightly upwards and represents the trunk of the artery. Its divisions can be marked as under:

  i. Anterior division
   - Mark the pterion by putting a point 4.5 cm above the mid-point of the zygomatic arch or by using *Stile's* method.
   - Mark the mid-point on the vertex between the inion and the nasion.

   Draw a line from the end of the trunk of the middle meningeal artery running upwards and slightly forwards to the first point with slight anterior convexity and then upwards and backwards in the direction of the second point. The frontal branch of the anterior division takes origin close to the pterion and passes upwards and forwards superficial to the motor speech centre of the left side.

  ii. Posterior division
   - Put a point on the upper limit of attachment of auricle.
   - Place a point on the lambda.

   Draw a line from the end of the trunk of the middle meningeal artery upwards and backwards towards the lambda through the first point.

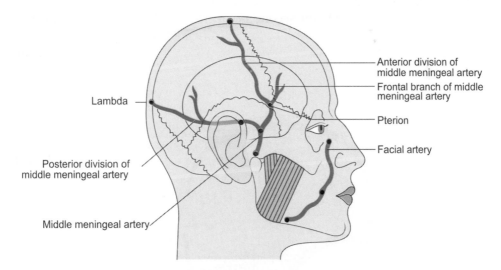

Fig. 5.7: Arteries of face

Veins and Sinuses

Anterior Facial Vein (Fig. 5.8)

- It is drawn just behind the location of the facial artery by taking similar points.

Cavernous Sinus

- It is on the medial side of the trigeminal ganglion (page 70) but extends to a more anterior position.

Sigmoid Sinus (Fig. 5.8)

- Put a point on the base of the mastoid process on the posterior aspect of the root of the external ear.
- Mark another point 1.2 cm above the mastoid tip.

Draw two lines 1.3 cm apart starting from the first point and going downwards along the line of reflection of the skin from the pinna to the head posteriorly and coming to the level of the lower margin of the meatus and then going forwards to the margin of the meatus which is opposite the jugular foramen.

Superior Sagittal Sinus (Fig. 5.8)

- Put a point on the glabella in the median plane.
- Mark the inion.

Draw a line upwards and backwards from the first point and continue it downwards and posteriorly to the second point. The line should be narrow in front and widen to about 1.2 cm at inion.

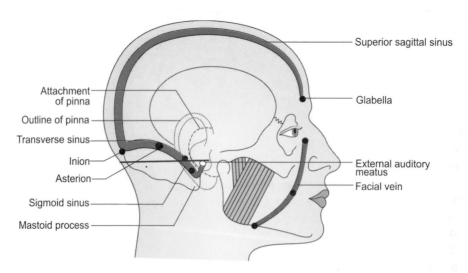

Fig. 5.8: Veins and venous sinuses of head

Transverse Sinus (Fig. 5.8)

- Put a point on the inion.
- Mark the asterion by a point 1.25 cm above a line drawn from the external auditary meatus to the external occipital protuberance and 3.75 cm behind the meatus.
- Place a point on the base of the mastoid process on the posterior aspect of the root of the external ear.

Draw the sinus by two lines 1.2 cm apart commencing at the inion and running laterally through the other points with a slight upwards convexity. The highest point will lie a little below the highest part of the external ear and will end on that portion of the mastoid process which lies behind the external ear.

NECK

SURFACE LANDMARKS (Figs 5.9 and 5.10)

- **Carotid tubercle** is on the transverse process of C 6 at the level of arch of cricoid cartilage, about 3 cm from the median plane behind the common carotid artery.
- **First rib:** The upper surface of the first rib has been outlined dotted. The trunks of brachial plexus can be palpated and rolled against it.

Median Line Landmarks of the Neck

By running a finger from the symphysis menti downwards the following can easily be felt in the order given below.

- Body of hyoid (level of C3). Greater cornu can be traced laterally.
- Laryngeal prominence (or Adam's apple). Thyroid cartilage lies at the level of C4 and C5.
- Arch of the cricoid cartilage lying at the level of C6.
- First ring of trachea.
- Isthmus of thyroid gland
- Supra-sternal notch.

- **Seventh cervical spine**. Can be palpated on the back of neck at the lower end of the nuchal furrow and is the first spine to be felt when the finger is run from above downwards (Fig. 5.2).
- **Sternomastoid muscle**. When the head is rotated to one side and tilted forwards, the muscle of the opposite side stands out and forms a visible landmark. The anterior border is seen extending from the sternum to the anterior border of mastoid process. The posterior border ascends from the junction of the medial and middle thirds of the clavicle to the mid-point between the mastoid process and inion.
- **Tip of the transverse process of atlas** lies midway between the tip of the mastoid process and the angle of mandible.

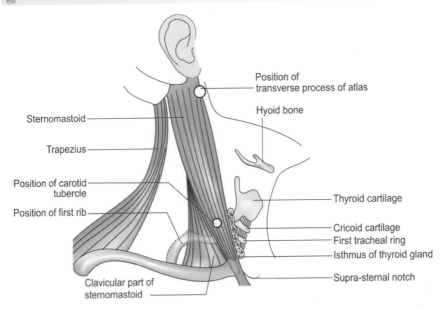

Position of
transverse process of atlas

Hyoid bone

Sternomastoid

Trapezius

Position of carotid
tubercle

Position of first rib

Thyroid cartilage

Cricoid cartilage
First tracheal ring
Isthmus of thyroid gland

Supra-sternal notch

Clavicular part of
sternomastoid

Fig. 5.9: Surface landmarks—neck

● **Trapezius.** Its anterior border can be seen when resistance is opposed to the elevation of the shoulder.

SURFACE MARKINGS

Gland

Thyroid Gland (Fig. 5.10)

  i. **Isthmus**
- Draw a line 1.5 cm long across the trachea, 1 cm below the arch of the cricoid cartilage to represent the upper border of isthmus.
- Draw another line 2 cm lower down to indicate the lower border of isthmus.

 ii. **Lateral lobes**
- Put a point 1 cm below the lateral end of the lower border of isthmus.
- Mark another point 2.5 cm below and lateral to the outer end of the lower border of isthmus.
- Put a point a little in front of the anterior border of sternomastoid at the level of laryngeal prominence to represent the extent of upper pole.

Lines joining the upper pole to the lateral end of the upper border of isthmus and to the lateral end of the lower pole complete the outline of the lateral lobe of the gland.

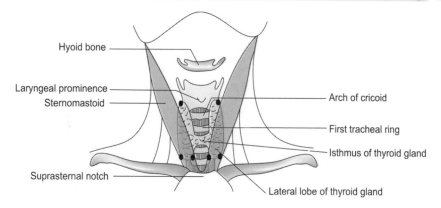

Fig. 5.10: Thyroid gland

Muscle

Scalenus Anterior (Fig. 5.13)

i. **Lateral border**
   - Put a point 2.5 cm from the median plane at the level of upper border of the thyroid cartilage.
   - Mark the junction of the medial and middle-third of the lower border of the clavicle.

   Join these points by a line running downwards and laterally.

ii. **Medial border**
   - Place a point 2.5 cm from the median plane at the level of the arch of the cricoid cartilage.
   - Put a point 1 cm medial to the lower end of the lateral border.

     Join these points by a line running downwards and laterally.

Nerves

Brachial Plexus (Fig. 5.11)

The upper limit is represented by a line drawn by joining the following points.
- The midpoint between the anterior and posterior borders of sternomastoid at the level of the cricoid cartilage.
- A point just external to the mid-point of the clavical.

Cervical Plexus

Anterior Cutaneous nerve of neck (Fig. 5.2)
- Mark the mid-point of the posterior border of sternomastoid.

Draw a line from this point across the muscle.

Great Auricular Nerve (Fig. 5.11)

- Put a point a little above the mid-point of the posterior border of sternomastoid. Draw a line from this point running upwards towards the lobule of the ear.

Lesser Occipital Nerve (Fig. 5.11)

- Put a point a little above the mid-point of the posterior border of sternomastoid. Draw a line from this point ascending along the posterior border of the muscle to reach the scalp.

Phrenic Nerve (Fig. 5.12)

- Put a point 3.5 cm from the median plane on a level with the upper border of thyroid cartilage.
- Put a point midway between the anterior and posterior borders of sternomastoid at the level of cricoid cartilage.
- Mark the sternal end of calvicle.
  Join these points to get the surface marking of the phrenic nerve.

Supra-clavicular Nerves (Fig. 5.11)

- Put a point a little below the mid-point of the posterior border of sternomastoid.
  Draw three lines descending towards the medial, intermediate and lateral-third of the clavicle.

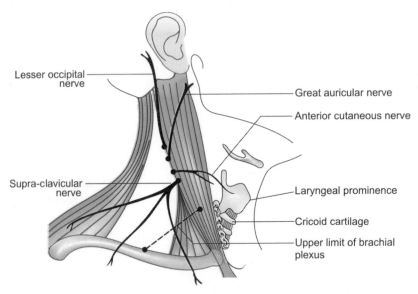

Fig. 5.11: Bronchial plexus and cutaneous nerves of neck

Cranial Nerves

Accessory Nerve (Fig. 5.12)

- Put a point on the lower and anterior part of the tragus.
- Mark the tip of the transverse process of the atlas.
- Put a point at the junction of the upper one-third and lower two-thirds of the posterior border of sternomastoid.
- Put a point on the anterior border of the trapezius, 6 cm above the clavicle.

Join these points by a line which goes downwards and backwards across the elevation produced by the sternomastoid and the depression of the posterior triangle of the neck.

Glossopharyngeal Nerve (Fig. 5.12)

- Put a point on the lower and anterior part of the tragus of ear.
- Mark a point just above the angle of mandible.

Join these points by a line which should continue along the lower border of mandible for a short while.

Hypoglossal Nerve (Fig. 5.12)

- Put a point on the lower and anterior part of tragus.
- Mark a point a little above and behind the tip of the greater cornu of the hyoid bone.

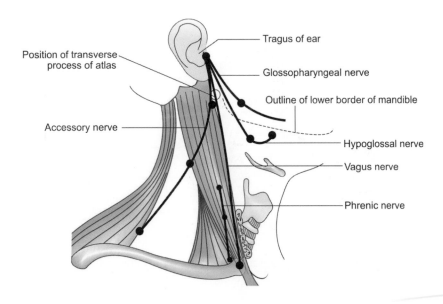

Fig. 5.12: Cranial nerves

- Put a point midway between the angle and symphysis of mandible with the head tilted backwards.

Join these points by a line which should bend sharply forwards and curve upwards between the second and third points.

Vagus Nerve (Fig. 5.12)

- Put a point on the lower and anterior part of the tragus.
- Mark the medial end of the clavicle.

Join these points to represent the nerve.

Sympathetic Trunk (Fig. 5.13)

- Place a point on the posterior border of the condyle of the mandible.
- Mark a point on the sterno-clavicular joint.

Join these points by a line to represent the trunk.

  i. *Superior cervical ganglion* is represented on this line by a spindle extending from transverse process of the atlas vertebra to the level of the greater cornu of the hyoid bone.

 ii. *Middle cervical ganglion* by a small circle opposite the arch of the cricoid cartilage

iii. *Inferior cervical ganglion* by a circle about 3 cm above the sterno-clavicular joint.

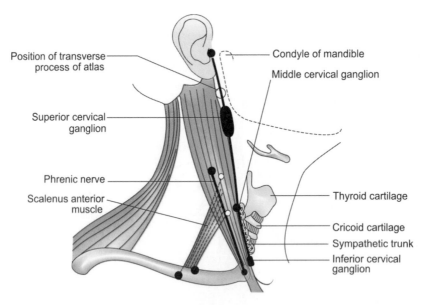

Fig. 5.13: Scalenus anterior nerve and sympathetic trunk

VESSELS

Arteries

Common Carotid Artery (Fig. 5.14)

- Mark the sterno-clavicular joint.
- Put a point on the anterior border of the sternomastoid at the level of upper border of thyroid cartilage.

  Join these points by double lines. (For thoracic part of left artery see page 38)

External Carotid Artery (Fig. 5.14)

- Put a point on the anterior border of sterno-mastoid at the level of the upper border of thyroid cartilage.
- Mark a point midway between the tip of the mastoid process and the angle of mandible.

  Join these points by double lines gently convex forwards in the lower half and gently convex backwards in the upper half.

Internal Carotid Artery (Fig. 5.14)

- Mark a point on the anterior border of sterno-mastoid at the level of the upper border of thyroid cartilage.
- Put a point at the posterior border of the condyle of mandible.

  Join these points by double lines.

Subclavian Artery (Fig. 5.14)

The following points should be marked with the shoulder well depressed.

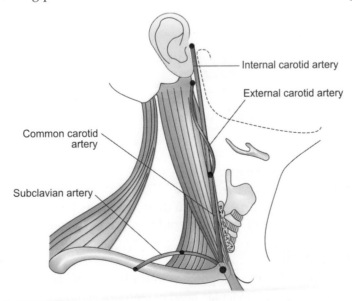

Fig. 5.14: Arteries of neck

- Mark the sterno-clavicular joint.
- Put a mark on the middle of the lower border of the clavicle.
- Mark another point 2 cm above the clavicle midway between the first and second points.

Join these points by a curved double line. (For thoracic part of left artery see page 38)

Veins

External Jugular Vein (Fig. 5.15)

- Place a point below the angle of the mandible.
- Mark another point on the upper border of the clavicle immediately lateral to the posterior border of sternomastoid muscle.

Draw a line downwards and backwards joining these points.

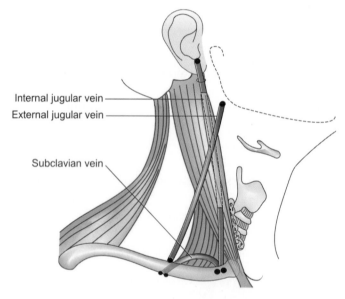

Fig. 5.15: Veins of neck

Internal Jugular Vein (Fig. 5.15)

- Put a point on the lobule of the ear.
- Mark the medial end of the clavicle.

Join these points by a double line making a dilatation at its lower end between the sternal and clavicular heads of sternomastoid to represent the inferior bulb.

Subclavian Vein (Fig. 5.15)

- Put a point a little medial to the midpoint of lower border of clavicle.
- Mark the medial edge of the clavicular head of sternomastoid.

Join these marks by a short double line convex upwards.

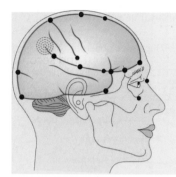

Brain

6

SURFACE LANDMARKS

These have been described with Head and Neck (see Chapter 5).

SURFACE MARKINGS

Cerebral Borders (Fig. 6.1)

Superciliary Border

- Place a point just above and lateral to the nasion.
- Mark another point a little above and a little lateral to the inion.
  Join these two points by a paramedian line.

Supermedial Border

- Put a point just above and lateral to the nasion.
- Place a point on the zygomatic process of frontal bone.
- Mark the pterion by a third point.
  Draw a line from the first point to arch upwards and laterally a little above the eyebrow to the second point and then to ascend to the third point.

Temporal Pole

- Put a point on the pterion.
- Place a point on the middle of the upper border of the zygomatic arch.
  Draw a line with the convexity forwards joining these points.

Infero-lateral Border

- Put a point on the middle of the upper border of the zygomatic arch.
- Mark another point just above and lateral to the inion.
  Draw a line backwards from the first point to cross the auricle a little above the external auditory meatus and then to descend slightly to the second point.

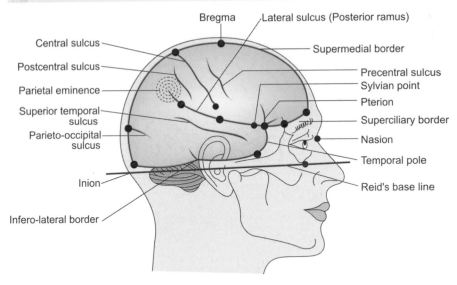

Fig. 6.1: Cerebrum—borders and sulci

CEREBRAL SULCI

Central Sulcus of Rolando (Fig. 6.1)

- Put a point 1.2 cm (a finger's breadth) behind the mid-point of the line joining the nasion to the inion in the median plane or a little less than 5 cm posterior to bregma.
- Mark a point 5 cm. vertically above the pre-auricular point (a thumb breadth behind the pterion).

Draw a line from the first point running downwards and laterally for about 8.75 cm with somewhat sinuous course and making an angle of 70° with the median plane as it joins the second point.

Precentral and Postcentral Sulci (Fig. 6.1)

- These are drawn parallel to the central sulcus 1.25 cm (a finger's breadth) in front and behind it respectively.

Lateral Sulcus (Fig. 6.1)

i. **Posterior ramus**
   - Put a point 4.5 cm above the middle point on zygomatic arch (Sylvian point)
   - Mark another point a finger's breadth above the top of the auricle.
   - Locate the parietal eminence and place a third point 1.2 cm below it.

Draw a line from the first point going backwards with an upward inclination to the second point. Curve the line sharply upwards to end at the parietal eminence.

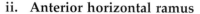

ii. **Anterior horizontal ramus**
     Draw a line 2 cm in length running horizontally forwards from the pterion.
iii. **Anterior ascending ramus**
     Draw a 2 cm long line running upwards from the pterion.
     Brocas area lies between these two anterior rami.

Superior Temporal Sulcus (Fig. 6.1)

Draw a line 1 cm below the posterior ramus of the lateral sulcus exhibiting a similar curve.

Parieto-occipital Sulcus (Fig. 6.1)

• Place a point about 1.2 cm in front of the lambda.
   Draw a line running lateralwards for about 2.5 cm from the longitudinal cerebral fissure at right angles from the above point.

CORTICAL AREAS

Motor Speech Centre of Broca (Fig. 6.2)

It is on the left side in right handed persons and on the right side in left handed ones and is situated between the two anterior rami of the lateral sulcus, immediately above and anterior to the Sylvian point, which is 4.5 cm above the middle point on the zygomatic arch.

It can also be roughly located by a finger tip placed immediately above the pterion on the left side (in the right handed people). Pterion can be located by the Stiles method as already described in page 67).

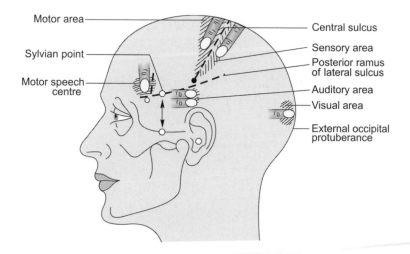

Fig. 6.2: Cortical functional areas

Motor Area (Fig. 6.2)

A strip, the breadth of a finger, laid in front of the line for the central sulcus would indicate its position.

Sensory Area (Fig. 6.2)

A strip, the breadth of a finger, placed immediately behind the line for the central sulcus would indicate its position.

Auditory Area (Fig. 6.2)

It is situated below the posterior part of the posterior ramus of lateral sulcus and lies roughly above the upper margin of the auricle.

Two finger tips placed side by side on the head a little above and in front of the top of the auricle are opposite the centre.

Visual Area (Fig. 6.2)

Most of it is situated on the medial side of the hemisphere; it becomes superficial posteriorly over a small area immediately above the external occipital protuberance.

Part II

Radiological Anatomy

 SUPERIOR EXTREMITY

 INFERIOR EXTREMITY

 BONE AGE

 THORAX

 ABDOMEN AND PELVIS

 HEAD AND NECK

 VERTEBRAL COLUMN

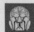 **ANGIOGRAPHY**

 NEW IMAGING DEVICES

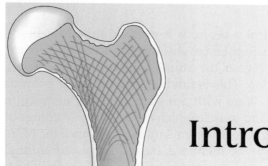

Introduction

INTRODUCTION (Fig. 1)

The study of anatomy by using X-rays is referred to as Radiological Anatomy. Many a fact in gross anatomy can be revealed and demonstrated in an X-ray plate (radiograph) and some of the organs (e.g. heart, diaphragm, stomach) may be seen functioning by looking into the screen on which shadows fall (fluoroscopy).

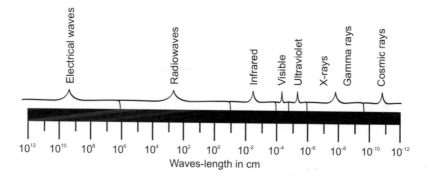

Fig. 1: Position of X-rays in electromagnetic radiations

Radiographs are an essential element in clinical diagnosis and a doctor has therefore to be well conversant with the anatomy of the normal radiograph of various regions before he can be proficient in the interpretation of complexities in disease.

X-rays were discovered by Wilhelm Konrad Rontgen, a German physicist, in 1895. They form a part of the spectrum of electromagnetic radiations, where the long electric and radio-waves are found at the one end; the infrared, visible, and ultra-violet light waves in the middle; and the X-rays, gamma rays and cosmic rays at the shortwave length end. It is thus apparent that the X-rays are of the same nature as light rays but have the distinguishing feature that their wavelengths are very short, 1/10000 of the wavelength of visible light. It is this characteristic that permits X-rays to penetrate materials which otherwise would absorb or reflect light.

Properties of X-rays

i. *Penetrating effect:* The penetration of a beam of X-rays is limited partly by scattering and partly by absorption. Substances absorb them according to their atomic weights and density; the higher the atomic weight or density of a substance, the greater the absorption. This is fundamental property as far as obtaining an image is concerned, Bone with a high percentage of calcium absorbs the X-rays more than skin and muscle which have a low percentage of calcium. The lower the atomic weights of the elements in a substance the more transparent will it be. Radiography is, therefore, based on the differential absorption of X-rays. Structures readily penetrated by X-rays are radiolucent; substances penetrated with difficulty or not at all are radiopaque.

ii. *Photographic effect:* X-rays affect photographic emulsions in much the same way as light. If a suitable type of photographic film is placed behind an object and an exposure made, the translucent parts allow the X-rays to pass through, so that these parts appear dark on the developed film. The dense parts absorb the X-rays, either partially or completely, and largely prevent them from reaching the film. In the corresponding parts of the film there is, therefore, less blackening effect so that when the film is viewed by transmitted white light a black and white picture is seen, the white parts corresponding to the dense parts in the object. This is known as a negative picture, and is in the form in which a skiagram (so called X-ray) is usually examined. Skiagram is therefore really a shadowgram (skia = shadow and gramma = a writing)

iii. *Fluorescent effect:* Light waves are produced if X-rays strike certain metallic salts (phosphorous). This is called fluorescence. Fluoroscopy or screening depends on this effect.

iv. *Biological effect:* X-rays can destroy abnormal cells (e.g., in malignant tumours) without destroying adjacent normal cells to the same degree. This is the basis of radiotherapy.

STANDARD VIEWS OF A RADIOGRAPH

Skiagrams are taken in different positions of the subject in relation to the source of X-ray! and the photographic film. Some of the common positions used are:

1. Antero-posterior view (AP)

It is taken with the X-ray tube anterior to the subject and the film posteriorly placed. Posterior structures are better visualised in this view.

2. Postero-anterior view (PA)

In this the X-ray tube is posterior to the subject and the film anterior, the rays thus passing postero-anteriorly through the subject. Anteriorly placed structures are more clearly visible in this view. The more commonly taken X-ray of the chest is a P.A. view.

3. Lateral views

These are used to assess the depth of the structures and can be:
  i.   *Right lateral view:* when the film is in contact with the right side of the subject,
  ii. *Left lateral view:* when the film is kept against the left side of the subject.

4. Oblique views

These are used for special study of a particular structure. In the case of chest X-rays these could be:
  i.   *Right anterior oblique view* (R.A.O)
  ii. *Left anterior oblique view* (L.A.O)
    The subject stands in front of upright film casette holder and is then turned 45° oblique (left or right).
    The orientation of a radiograph is marked by incorporating a lead letter into the cassette before exposing a film, e.g. the right side with an 'R', and left side with an 'L'.

TYPES OF RADIOGRAPHS

1. Plain Radiographs

When X-rays are allowed to pass through the subject without the use of any medium the translucent portions appear black on the developed X-ray plate, whereas the dense areas absorb the X-rays in varying degrees resulting in different shades of white.

2. Contrast Radiographs

When X-rays are taken after filling a cavity or space with a contrast medium in order to visualise the lumen of the viscus or extent of the cavity.
    The contrast media are of two types:
  a. *Opaque,* e.g. barium sulphate for the gastro-intestinal tract, and iodine compounds for the urinary tract.
  b. *Translucent,* e.g. air or oxygen for ventricles of brain.

X-RAY APPEARANCES OF NORMAL SKELETON (Fig. 2)

Structure of Mature Bone

Because of their high calcium content, the bones of the skeleton are clearly defined and contrasted with the soft parts. The long bones show a dense white homogenous outer layer, the cortex, which encloses a less dense inner portion, the cancellous bone, which is represented by a series of fine white lines that correspond to the thin sheets of bone known as the trabeculae or lamellae. These lamellae are arranged mainly in the direction of the predominant stress, but are joined to each other by cross bracing lamellae. Lamellae placed on the lines of pressure are seen particularly clearly, in the neck of the femur (calcar-femorale) and in the calcaneum, because

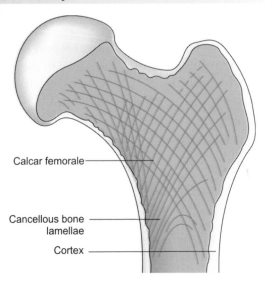

Calcar femorale

Cancellous bone
lamellae

Cortex

Fig. 2: Structure of mature bone

they are subjected to great stress.In the long bones of the limbs generally they tend to run vertically, but the number of cross bracing obscures the pattern. Study of the trabecular architecture and the distribution of the cortical and cancellous layers in each bone is useful because alterations occur in many pathological conditons.

In the shafts of the long bones the cancellous bone is absent and is replaced by a space, the medullary (marrow) cavity, which can be seen in a skiagram though its limits are not clearly demarcated.

Structure of Immature Bone

At birth considerable portions of the skeleton are formed of cartilage, the radiographic density of which is much the same as that of the overlying skin and muscles. These portions are therefore not normally distinguished in a skiagram e.g. the cartilaginous carpal elements in the wrist and the ends of certain long bones of the extremities.

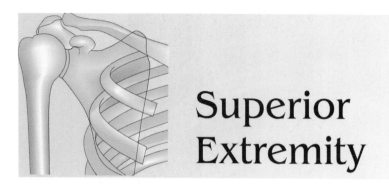

Superior Extremity

7

SHOULDER REGION

RADIOGRAPHIC APPEARANCE

Antero-posterior View (Fig. 7.1)

When an antero-posterior view is taken with the arm by the side the following details are noticed.

- **Acromio-clavicular joint** as a gap between the clavicle and the acromion.
- **Acromion** lying partly behind the head of humerus and superimposed on it.
- **Anatomical neck of humerus:** Medial portion is on a level with the junction of the middle and lower thirds of the glenoid cavity. It appears as an angular notch.
- **Clavicle.** Lateral half of the clavicle projects a little higher than the adjacent upper surface of the acromion.
- **Conoid tubercle** as a bony prominence on the inferior surface of the clavicle near the outer third.
- **Coracoid process** as a more or less circular shadow below the lateral third of the clavicle.
- **Glenoid cavity** as a narrow ellipse.
- **Greater tuberosity of humerus** as the most lateral bony point in the shoulder region.
- **Head of the humerus** lying against the glenoid cavity.
- **Inferior angle of scapula** is seen partly superimposed on the lung field, at the level of the seventh rib or seventh intercostal space.
- **Lesser tuberosity and bicipital groove** are difficult to identify.
- **Superior angle of scapula** projects upwards in the angle between the clavicle and the first rib.

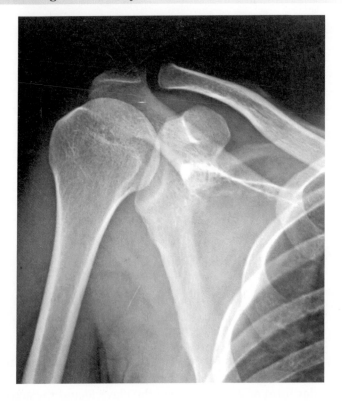

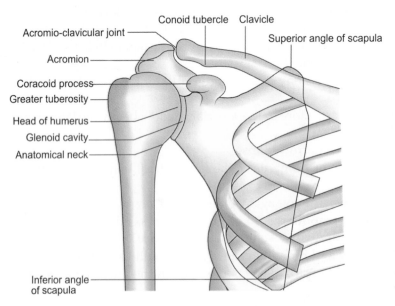

Fig. 7.1: Shoulder—AP view

ELBOW

RADIOGRAPHIC APPEARANCE

Antero-Posterior View (Fig. 7.2)

With fully extended elbow shows the following:

- **Elbow joint space** as a translucent broad line passing across the ulna between the trochlea and coronoid process. It separates the head of the radius from the capitulum.
- **Head and tuberosity of radius** is seen slightly overlapping the ulna.
- **Lateral epicondyle of humerus** gives a flatter appearance as compared to the medial epicondyle.
- **Medial epicondyle of humerus** is seen projecting medially.
- **Olecranon process** is superimposed on the shadow of the humerus and its proximal limit can be recognised below the shadow cast by the **Coronoid and olecranon fossae**.
- **Trochlea** is superimposed by ulna.

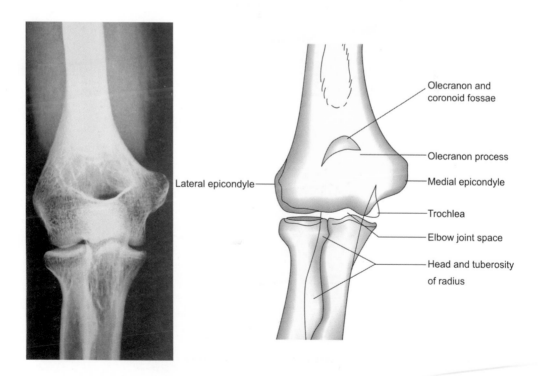

Fig. 7.2: Elbow—AP view

Lateral View (Fig. 7.3)

In right angle flexion the special features to be noted are:

- **Capitulum** is seen projecting anteriorly beyond the line of the anterior edge of the shaft of the humerus.
- **Coronoid process** partly overlaps the shadow of the head of the radius.
- **Epicondyles.** The shadows of lateral and medial epicondyles are superimposed.
- **Head of the radius** lies opposite the capitulum.
- **Olecranon process** is seen projecting backwards.
- **Supracondylar ridges** are seen as white lines passing upwards from the epicondylar shadows.

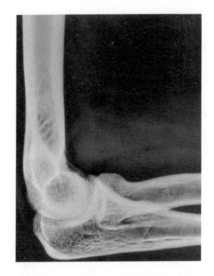

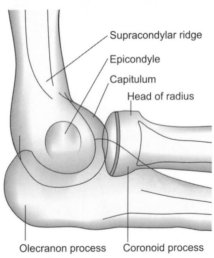

Fig. 7.3: Elbow—lateral view

WRIST AND HAND

RADIOGRAPHIC APPEARANCE

Postero-Anterior View (Fig. 7.4)

● **Carpal bones** can be easily recognised. From lateral to medial side. They are:
  i. *Proximal row*— scaphoid, lunate, triquetral and pisiform.
     Pisiform shadow is superimposed on that of the triquetral.
  ii. *Distal row* —trapezium, trapezoid, capitate and hamate.
     Hook of hamate appears as on oval white ring.
     Trapezium and trapezoid slightly overlap each other.

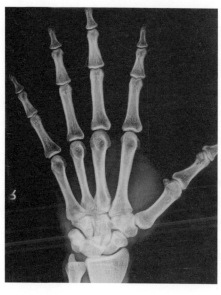

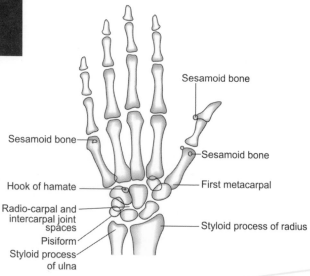

Fig. 7.4: Wrist and hand—AP view

Metacarpals

First lies somewhat laterally on the trapezium. It is seen obliquely and slightly distorted. *Second, third, fourth* and *fifth* outline of each is easily defined. The bases tend to overlap.

- **Phalanges** are seen separated by interphalangeal joints. The terminal phalanges give a spade like appearance.
- **Radio-carpal and inter-carpal joint spaces** are clearly seen.
- **Radio-ulnar joint space** is mostly obscured by overlapping bones.
- **Sesamoid bones:** In the hand the following sesamoid bones are of almost constant occurrence.
    i. Two opposite the head of the first metacarpal in the tendon of flexor pollicis brevis muscle.
    ii. One sesamoid bone is also sometimes seen opposite the head of the fifth metacarpal.
    iii. One or two sesamoid bones are frequently present opposite the interphalangeal joint of the thumb, they lie in the flexor tendons.
- **Styloid process of radius and ulna:** The styloid process of radius extends further distally than that of ulna.

Inferior Extremity

8

THE HIP REGION

RADIOGRAPHIC APPEARANCE

Antero-posterior View (Fig. 8.1)

The patient is placed flat on his back with the toe of his foot pointing somewhat to the median plane. This later measure is of importance so that the neck of the femur is not foreshortened.

- **Acetabulum:** The superior and medial edge appears as a curved white line of cortical bone. The posterior rim is seen partly superimposed on the head of the femur.
- **Greater trochanter:** In anatomical position of the foot, it lies in a plane somewhat posterior to the head of the femur. In external rotation its shadow overlaps that of the head. The contour of the greater trochanter tends to be poorly defined in a usual X-ray of hip region.
- **Head of femur:** The cortex of the head of femur casts a white line. Fovea capitis femoris is visible as a small depression on the head.
- **Hip joint space** appears as a radiolucent interval between the white lines of the rim of acetabulum and the head of the femur.
- **Lesser trochanter:** Its situation is of interest because the extent to which it is visible affords a rough guide to the position of the limb at the time of exposure. It appears as a more prominent projection when the femur is laterally rotated than when it is medially rotated.
- **Neck of femur:** The neck of the femur as seen in Fig. 8.1 normally makes an angle of 25°–30° to the coronal plane. The femoral head projects medially and markedly forwards.

The neck of the femur has a relatively constant angle with the shaft which is usually between 120 and 140 degrees, being more in children and less in females, who have a wider pelvis.

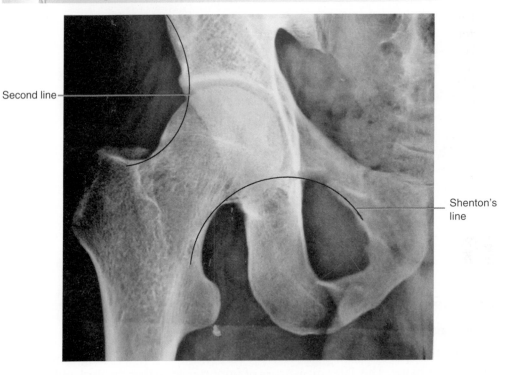

Second line

Shenton's line

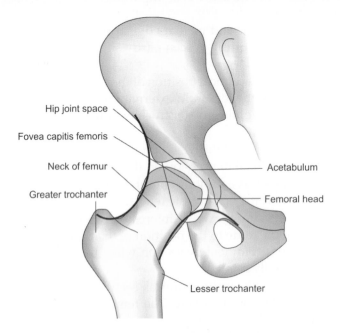

Hip joint space

Fovea capitis femoris

Neck of femur

Greater trochanter

Acetabulum

Femoral head

Lesser trochanter

Fig. 8.1: Hip—AP view

The pressure lamellae in the femoral neck (calcar femorale) have a distinctive pattern (Fig. 8.2).

The periphery of the normal femoral neck and the pelvic bone produce two regular curvatures, the appreciation of which are of considerable value in recognising displacements.

(i) **Shenton's line:** The line of the upper margin of the obturator foramen follows the same curve as that of the under surface of the neck and medial side of the shaft of the femur (lower line on X-ray plate).

(ii) **The second line:** It is indicated as forming the lateral border of the ilium from the anterior-superior iliac spine across the hip joint and continued on to the superior border of the femoral neck and to the greater trochanter (upper line on X-ray plate).

 KNEE

RADIOGRAPHIC APPEARANCE

Antero-posterior View (Fig. 8.2)

In antero-posterior view taken in full extension the following features should be noted:

- **Articular ends of femur and tibia** are demarcated by thin white lines of cortical bone.
- **Head and styloid process of the fibula** are seen considerably below the knee joint space on the lateral side and are superimposed by tibia.

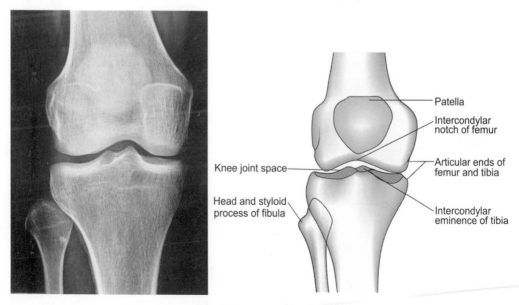

Fig. 8.2: Knee—AP view

- **Intercondylar eminence of tibia** presents a spinous appearance on the middle of the upper surface of tibia.
- **Intercondylar notch of femur** is variable and superimposed by patella.
- **Knee joint space** is normally a 0.5 cm gap cast due to the radiolucency of the articular cartilages.
- **Patella** is superimposed on the lower end of femur and appears as a more or less circular translucent shadow with the lower edge lying about 1.25 cm above the knee joint space.

Lateral View (Fig. 8.3)

The knee is partially flexed, and its lateral aspect placed next to film.

- **Intercondylar eminence of tibia** is slightly overlapped by the femoral condyles. The spine lies somewhat behind the midpoint of the superior surface of tibial condyles.
- **Knee joint space** is obscured by the overlappping bone shadows.
- **Medial and lateral femoral condyles:** The anterior and posterior margins of two condyles are not superimposed due to the difference in their diameters.
- **Patella** is seen in front of the condyles of femur.

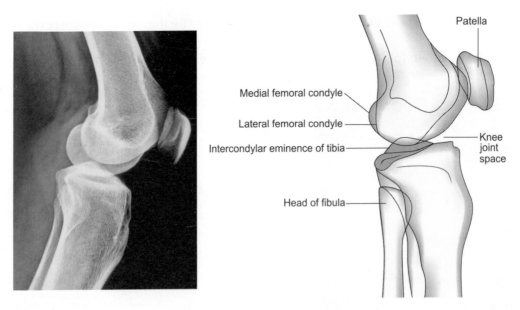

Medial femoral condyle

Lateral femoral condyle

Intercondylar eminence of tibia

Head of fibula

Patella

Knee joint space

Fig. 8.3: Knee—lateral view

ANKLE

RADIOGRAPHIC APPEARANCE

Antero-posterior View (Fig. 8.4)

● **Lower end of fibula** is superimposed on the tibia. The joint space between it and the talus is not visible in this view.

● **Lower end of tibia** is seen separated from the upper surface of talus by the ankle joint space which is continued on the medial side of talus and separates the same from the medial malleolus.

● **Talus** casts a four-sided shadow below the lower ends of tibia and fibula.

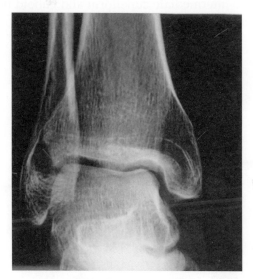

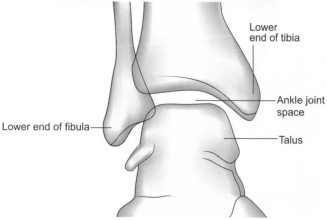

Fig. 8.4: Ankle—AP view

FOOT

RADIOGRAPHIC APPEARANCE

Antero-posterior View (Fig. 8.5)

In this position the sole is on the film.

The outline of various tarsal and metatarsal bones and phalanges can be clearly made out.

● **Calcaneum:** Its anterior part can be easily made out.
● **Cuboid bone** articulates directly with calcaneum on its proximal surface.
● **Cuneiform bones** medial, intermediate and lateral can be seen articulating with the navicular proximally. The lateral cuneiform presents an obscure outline by overlapping with the intermediate cuneiform and cuboid bones.
● **Intertarsal joint spaces** are clearly visible.

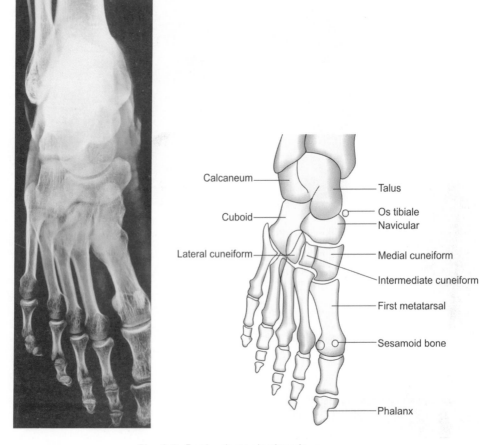

Fig. 8.5: Foot—dorsoplantar view

● **Metatarsals** are seen articulating with the distal row of tarsal bones. The outline of each is easily defined. The body of the first metatarsal is heavy, but the bodies of the remainder are slender. The bases tend to overlap.

● **Navicular** is an additional element between the two rows of tarsal bones and is interposed between the talus of proximal row and the medial three bones of the distal row.

● **Phalanges** are seen separated by the interphalangeal joints.

● **Talus:** Its posterior part cannot be made out clearly.

● **Tarsal bones**
  i. *Proximal row of tarsal bones* is comprised of talus and calcaneum which do not lie side by side but are placed one above the other.
  ii. *Distal row comprises of four bones.* Named from the medial side to the lateral side, they are medial cuneiform, intermediate cuneiform, lateral cuneiform and cuboid. These bones are seen lying side by side.

● **Sesamoid bones:** Prominent medial and lateral sesamoid bones are usually seen to overlap the head of the first metatarsal bone.

● **Supernumerary bones:** There are three common ones.
  i. *Os tibiale* lies close to the tuberosity of navicular (Fig. 8.5)
  ii. *Os trigonum* lies at the posterior end of the talus (Fig. 8.6)
  iii. *Os peronei* is a sesamoid bone in the tendon of peroneus longus and lies close to the cuboid (Fig. 8.6).

Lateral View of the Ankle and Foot (Fig. 8.6)

In this position the lateral malleolus is on the film.

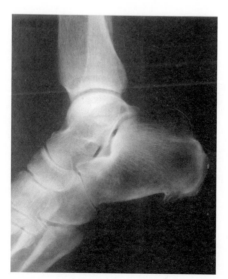
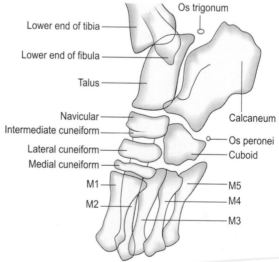

Fig. 8.6: Ankle and foot—lateral view

- **Calcaneum:** It is seen projecting backwards. The pressure lamellae in the calcaneum present their characteristic pattern.
- Cuboid shows its prominent pojecting ridge on the plantar outline.
- **Cuneiforms:** These three bones are superimposed and their position can be decided by recognising trio cuneiform-metatarsal joint spaces.
- **Lower end of fibula:** It is seen partly superimposed on the tibia and talus. The shadow of the lateral malleolus is lower than that of the medial malleolus.
- **Metatarsals:** The first (M_1), second (M_2) and third (M_3) tend to be partly superimposed. The fourth can be clearly demarcated (M_4). The fifth (M_5) has the tubercle on its base.
- **Navicular** is easily identified anterior to the head of the talus.
- **Talus** is seen mounted on the calcaneum and is itself ridden over by the lower end of tibia.
- **Lower end of tibia** is easily made out and the talo-tibial joint space is clearly visible. The medial malleolus overlaps the talus.

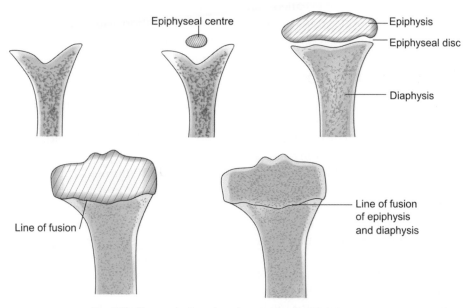

Bone Age

SKELETAL MATURATION (Fig. 9.1)

In early foetal life, a long bone is preceded by a model of hyaline cartilage. The areas where the bone formation or ossifications start in the cartilaginous model are known as centres of ossification. These centres may be primary or secondary. As a rule primary centres appear before birth and the secondary centres after birth. A typical long bone ossifies in three parts, the two ends from secondary centres and the intervening shaft from a primary centre.

Fig. 9.1: Stages in the development of a long bone

The secondary centres are also known as epiphyseal centres of ossification and the age at which they first become visible on a skiagram is known as the date of appearance of the epiphysis. These epiphyseal centres appear at different ages in different parts of the skeleton. In early stages of ossification, an epiphysis appears as an irregular nodule on the skiagram. Sometimes ossification starts from several centres simultaneously, as in the patella, but these soon merge into a single bony mass.

The epiphyseal ossification spreads and gradually replaces the cartilaginous epiphysis except where it is adjacent to diaphysis. The cartilage which persists between the epiphysis and the diaphysis is known as the epiphyseal disc. It appears as a narrow translucent band in a skiagram. The cartilage of this disc grows and is progressively replaced by bone which is added to the end of the diaphysis. Growth in length of the bone ceases when the cells of the cartilage cease to multiply, bone from the metaphysis then extends across the epiphyseal disc. Osseous contiguity is thus established between the epiphyseal and the diaphyseal ossification. This is known as the "fusion of the epiphysis" in radiological terms. The bone formed at the site of epiphyseal disc is particularly dense and is recognisable on the radiographs of young and even middle-aged adults. Knowledge of this prevents confusion with fracture lines.

The growing skeleton is sensitive to relatively slight and transient illnesses and to periods of malnutrition. Proliferation of cartilage at the metaphysis slows down during starvation and illness, but degeneration of cartilage cells in the columns continues, producing a dense line of provisional calcification which later becomes bone with thicker trabeculae called "lines of arrested growth" as seen in X-rays.

In some cases of endocrinopathy, chromosomal aberration, Morquio's syndrome, or dyschondroplasia, whole group of ossification centres may fail to appear.

PRINCIPLES OF OSSIFICATION

1. The primary centres appear before birth (usually between seventh and twelfth week) with some exception. The primary centres of tarsal and carpal bones appear after birth, excepting those of talus, calcaneum and cuboid.
2. The secondary or epiphyseal centres appear, as a rule, after birth (usually from the time of birth to five years of age) excepting at the lower end of femur, and sometimes at the upper end of the tibia and the upper end of humerus.
3. The development of short bones is similar to that of the primary centres of long bones and only one the calcaneum, develops a secondary centre of ossification.
4. In long bones with two epiphyses, the epiphysis whose centre of ossification appears first is usually the last to fuse with the shaft. The fibula is an exception to this rule. The centre for the head appears later than that for the distal end, but fuses later. The centre appears first in the lower end because it is a pressure epiphysis. The delay in fusion of the upper end may be associated with more prolonged growth at the knee (growing end).

5. In long bones with a single epiphysis, that epiphysis is at the more movable end. Thus in metacarpals, metatarsals and phalanges, these epiphyses include the heads of metacarpals and metatarsals 2 to 5, and the bases of the first metacarpal and metatarsal and the bases of all the phalanges.

6. The epiphyseal centre of ossification appears earliest in the largest of the epiphysis of a long bone.

7. When epiphysis forms from more than one centre (e.g. proximal end of humerus) the various centres coalesce before union occurs with the diaphysis.

8. From twelve or fourteen years to twentyfive years epiphyses fuse with the diaphyses, and growth ceases as fusion occurs.

9. In general, the appearance of epiphyseal centres and their fusion occur about one year earlier in females than in males so that the female skeleton matures more rapidly than the male. The longer period of growth in the male accounts partly for the average greater size of the male adult, just as the earlier start in the female accounts for the greater size of the average girl until the teenage is reached.

"BONE AGE" ESTIMATION

The age of a growing skeleton may be fairly reliably estimated since the appearance and union of the centres of ossification occur in a fairly definite pattern and time sequence from birth to maturity. Roentgenologic study of osseous development provides a valuable guide for evaluation of normal and abnormal growth. The skeletal maturity of any individual is known as the 'bone age'. A radiologist determines the bone age of a person by assessing ossification centres. Two criteria are used.

i. The number and size of epiphyseal centres demonstrable at a given chronological age. The time of appearance is specific for each epiphysis of each bone for each sex. Thus the principles governing their sequence and their site of appearance should be known

ii. The disappearance of the dark line representing the epiphyseal cartilage plate which indicates that the epiphysis has fused to the diaphysis. The sequence of dates of union is remarkably constant and the intervals between them remain proportionately the same in different people.

Students are no longer required to memorize long lists of dates as these can always be referred to in a book, but it is important in radiographs of the young and adolescent to be able to recognise the sites of epiphyseal lines in order to distinguish them from fracture lines. Traumatic separation of the epiphysis from the diaphysis may sometimes occur, e.g. the medial epicondyle of the humerus.

The chronological order of appearance of ossification centres and of union of epiphysis with diaphysis have been summarised in Tables 9.1 to 9.3.

Dates given for individual bones in this text are approximations based on those given in Grays Textbook of Anatomy.

For convenience, figures for the male are given. In females, they are about one to two years earlier as mentioned before.

SUPERIOR EXTREMITY

Sequence of Ossification and Union at the Shoulder (Figs 9.2a to f)

Appearance
1st year   – Head of humerus
2nd year – Greater tuberosity
5th year   – Lesser tuberosity (not visible)
6th year   – Fusion of the epiphyses of upper end of humerus into one mass.

Fusion

20th year – Fusion of upper end of humerus with shaft.

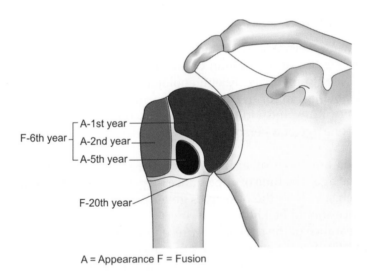

F-6th year ┤ A-1st year
           A-2nd year
           A-5th year

F-20th year

A = Appearance F = Fusion

Fig. 9.2a: Shoulder—ossification and union

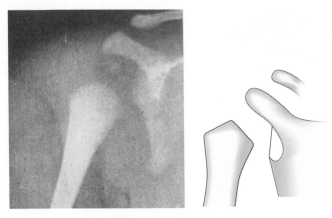

Fig. 9.2b: At birth epiphysis head humerus absent

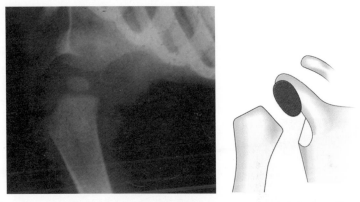

Fig. 9.2c: Age above 1 year (epiph head humerus present) below 2 years (epiph. gt. tub. absent)

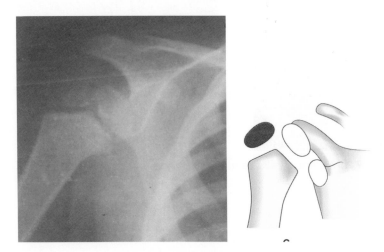

Fig. 9.2d: Age above 2 years (epiph. gt. tub. present) below 6 years (epiph. head and gt. tub. not fused)

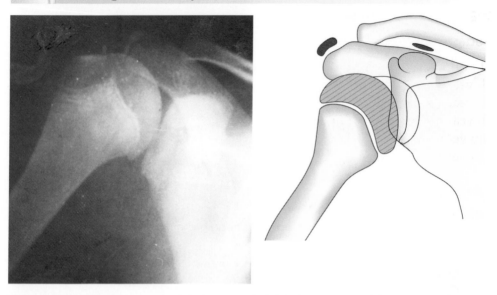

Fig. 9.2e: Age above 6 years (epiph. head and gt. tub, fused) below 20 years (epiph not fused with shaft)

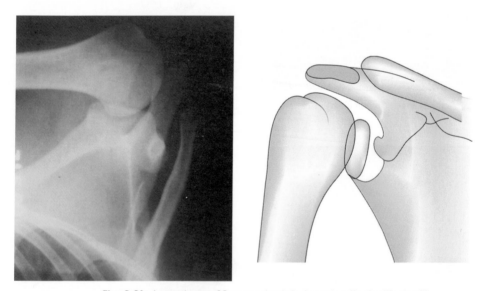

Fig. 9.2f: Age above 20 years (epiph. head united with shaft)

SEQUENCE OF OSSIFICATION AND UNION AT THE ELBOW (Figs 9.3a to h)

Appearance

1st year	–	Capitulum and lateral part of trochlea.
5th year	–	Head of radius.
6th year	–	Medial epicondyle of humerus.
9th year	–	Medial part of trochlea.
10th year	–	Top of olecranon process.
12th year	–	Lateral epicondyle of humerus.

Fusion

15th year	–	Fusion of olecranon epiphysis with upper end of ulna.
16th year	–	Fusion of lateral epicondyle, capitulum and trochlea into one mass.
	–	Fusion of capitulum, trochlea and lateral epicondyle to shaft.
17th year	–	Fusion of head of radius to shaft.
20th year	–	Fusion of medial epicondyle of humerus to shaft.

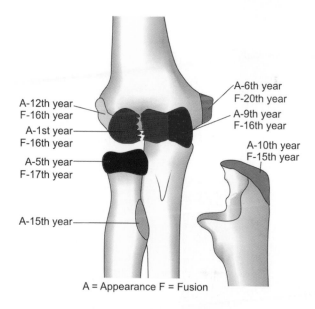

A = Appearance F = Fusion

Fig. 9.3a: Elbow—ossification and union

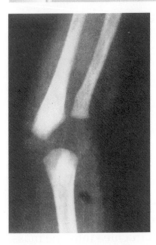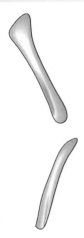

Fig. 9.3b: A birth (epiph. absent)

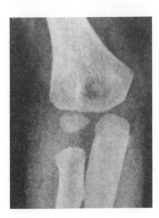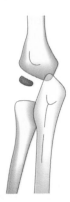

Fig. 9.3c: Age above 1 year (epiph. capitulum and lat trochlea present) below 5 years (epiph. head radius absent)

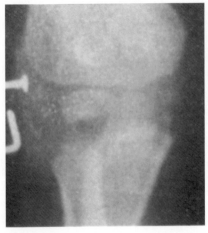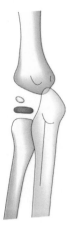

Fig. 9.3d: Age above 5 years (epiph. head radius present) below 6 years (epiph. med. epicondyle absent)

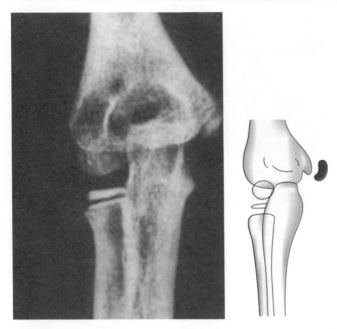

Fig. 9.3e: Age above 6 years (epiph, med. epicondyle present) below 10 years (epiph. med. trochlea absent)

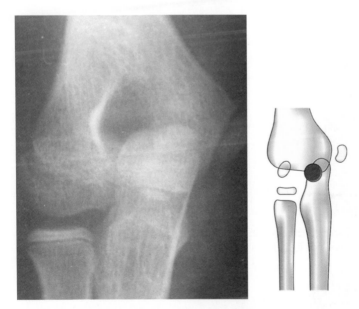

Fig. 9.3f: Age above 10 years (epiph. med. trochlea present) below 12 years (epiph. lat. epicondyle absent)

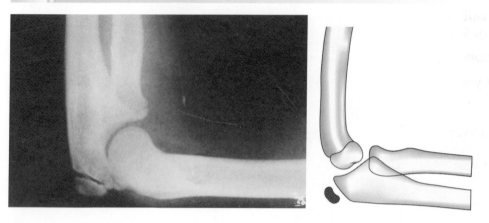

Fig. 9.3g: Age above 11 years (epiph top olecranon present) below 15 years (epiph. olecranon not fused with shaft)

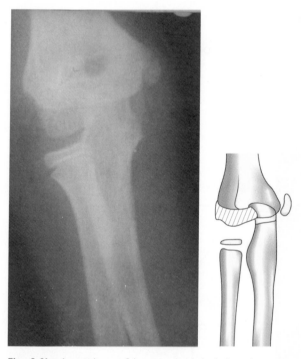

Fig. 9.3h: Age above 16 years (epiph. lat. epicond. capitulum and trochlea fused to shaft) below 17 years (epiph. head radius not fused to shaft)

SEQUENCE OF OSSIFICATION AND UNION AT THE HAND AND THE WRIST
(Figs 9.4a to j)

Appearance

1st year	– Lower end of radius
	– Capitate
	– Hamate
2nd year	– Heads of second, third, fourth and fifth metacarpals
	– Bases of the proximal phalanges
3rd year	– Triquetral
	– Base of the first matacarpal
	– Base of middle phalanges
	– Base of terminal phalanges
4th year	– Lunate
5th year	– Scaphoid
	– Trapezium
	– Trapezoid
6th year	– Lower end of ulna
12th year	– Pisiform

Fusion

17th year	– Fusion of the base of first metacarpal
18th year	– Fusion of the epiphysis of metacarpals and phalanges
	– Fusion of the lower end of ulna
19th year	– Fusion of the lower end of radius

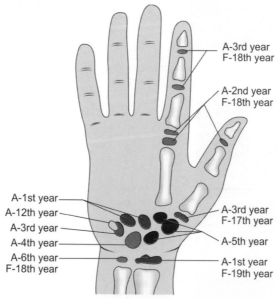

A = Appearance F = Fusion

Fig. 9.4a: Hand and wrist—ossification and union

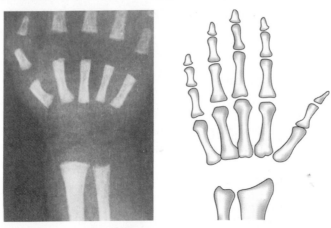

Fig. 9.4b: At birth (no carpal bone ossified)

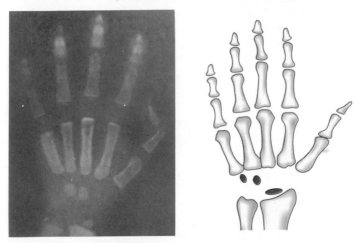

Fig. 9.4c: Age above 1 year (Capitate, hamate and epiph. lower end radius present) below 2 years (epiph 2nd to 5th metacarp. heads absent)

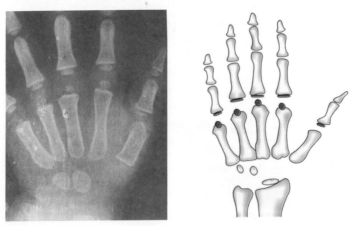

Fig. 9.4d: Age above 2 years (epiph. 2nd to 5th metacarp. heads and bases prox. phalanges present) below 3 years (ossif. centre triquetral and 1st metacap. base absent)

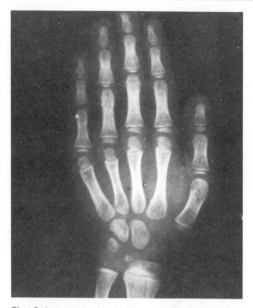 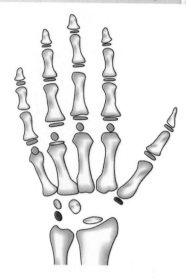

Fig. 9.4e: Age above 3 years (triquetral and epiph. 1st metacarp base present) below 4 years (ossif. centre lunate absent)

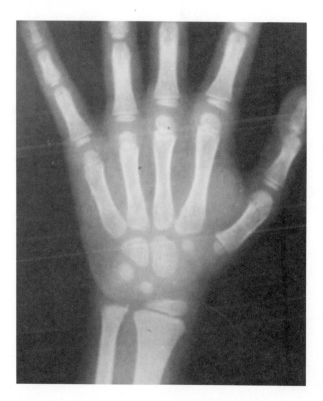 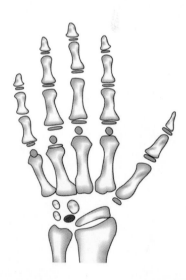

Fig. 9.4f: Age above 4 years (lunate present) below 5 years (ossif. centres scaphoid, trapezium and trapezoid absent)

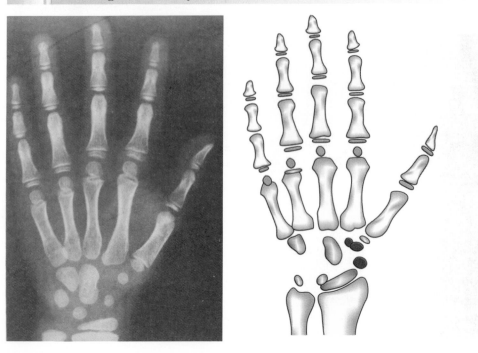

Fig. 9.4g: Age above 5 years (scaphoid, trapezium and trapezoid present) below 6 years (epiph. lower end ulna absent)

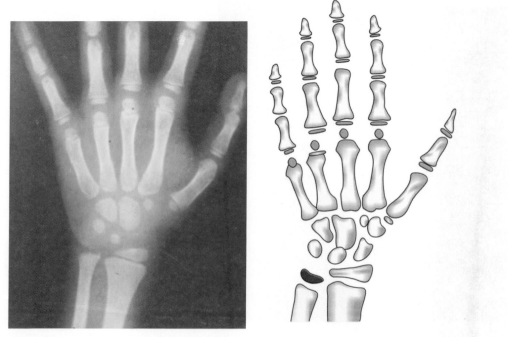

Fig. 9.4h: Age above 6 years (epiph. lower end ulna present) below 12 years, cossif. centre pisiform absent)

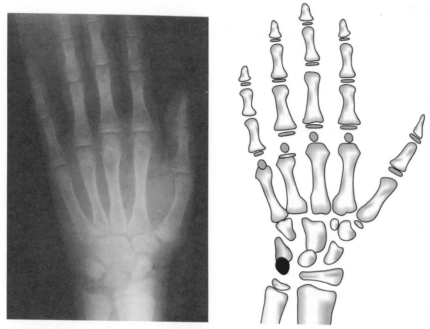

Fig. 9.4i: Age above 12 years (pisiform present) below 17 years (epiph base of first metacarp not fused)

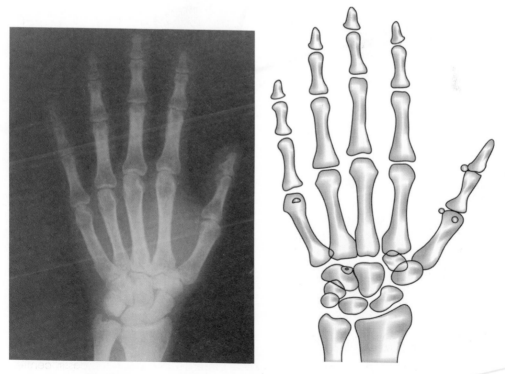

Fig. 9.4j: Age above 19 years (epiph lower end of radius fused)

INFERIOR EXTREMITY

Sequence of Ossification and Union at the Hip Region (Figs 9.5a to g)

Appearance

1st year—Head of femur.
4th year—Greater trochanter.
8th year—Fusion of the inferior ramus of the pubis with the ramus of ischium
12th to 14th year—Lesser trochanter.

Fusion
15th year—Lesser trochanter.
16th year—Greater trochanter.
17th year—Head of femur with shaft.
20th to 25th year—Disappearance of acetabular triradiate cartilage to fuse the three parts of hip bone.

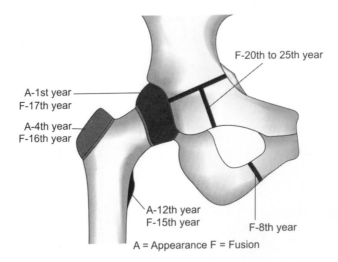

Fig. 9.5a: Hip—ossification and union

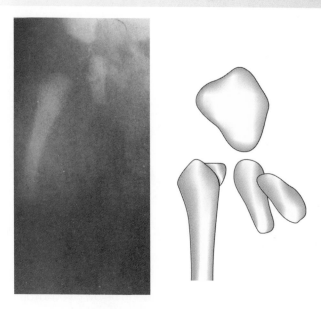

Fig. 9.5b: At birth (epiph. head femur absent)

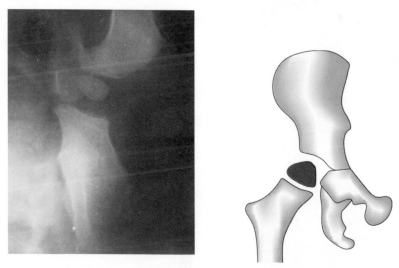

Fig. 9.5c: Age above 1 year (epiph. head femur present) below 4 years (epiph. gt. trochanter absent)

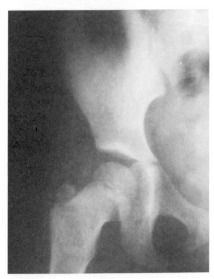
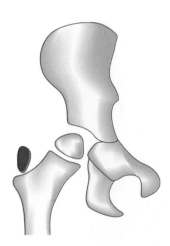

Fig. 9.5d: Age above 4 years (epiph. gt. trochanter present) below 8 years (rami of pubis and ischium not fused)

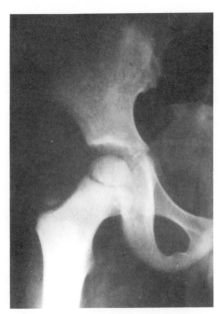
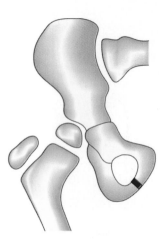

Fig. 9.5e: Age above 8 years (rami of pubis and ischium fused) below 16 years (epiph. gt. trochanter not fused with shaft.)

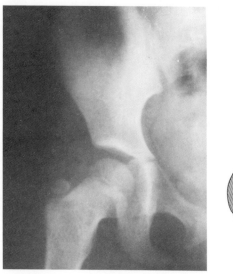
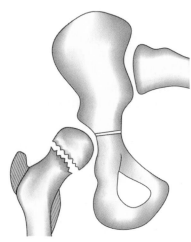

Fig. 9.5f: Age above 16 years (epjph. gt. trochanter fused with shaft) below 17 years (epiph. head femur not fused with shaft)

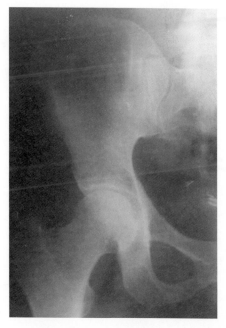
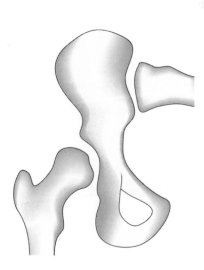

Fig. 9.5g: Age above 20 years (fusion of three parts of hip bone at acetabulum)

Sequence of Ossification and Union at the Knee (Figs 9.6a to h)

Appearance

Present at birth—Lower end of femur
1st year—Upper end of tibia (may be present at birth)
3rd to 6th year—Patella
4th year—Upper end of fibula
10th year—Tongue-like extension of tibial epiphysis for tibial tubercle.

Fusion

18th year	Lower end of femur with shaft.
	Upper end of tibia with shaft.
19th year	Upper end of fibula with shaft.

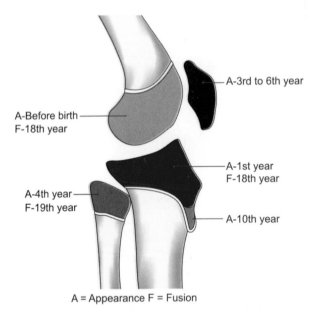

A = Appearance F = Fusion

Fig. 9.6a: Knee—ossification and union

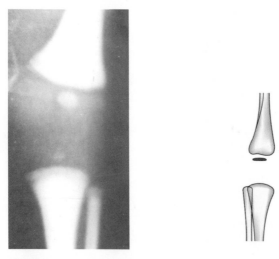

Fig. 9.6b: At birth (epiph. lower end femur present and upper end tibia may also be present)

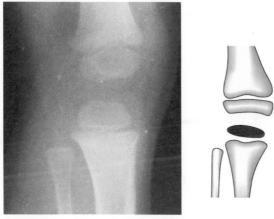

Fig. 9.6c: Age above 1 year (epiph. upper end tibia present) below 4 years (epioh. upper end fibula absent)

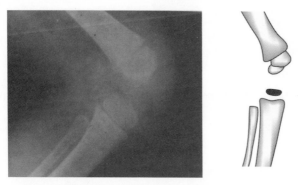

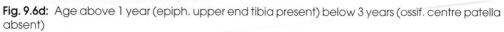

Fig. 9.6d: Age above 1 year (epiph. upper end tibia present) below 3 years (ossif. centre patella absent)

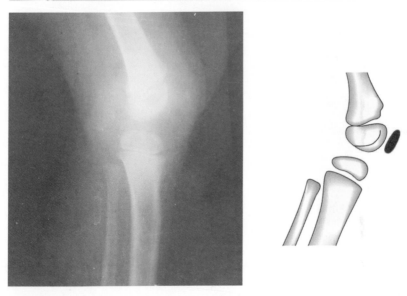

Fig. 9.6e: Age above 3 years (Ossif, centre patella present) below 4 years (epiph, upper end fibula absent)

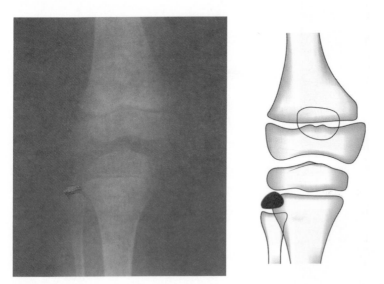

Fig. 9.6f: Age above 4 years (epiph. upper end fibural present, below 18 years (epiph.femur and tibia not used with shaft)

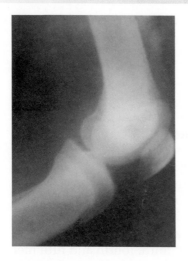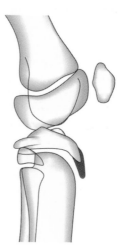

Fig. 9.6g: Age above 10 yrs (epiph, tibial tub. present) below 18 yrs (epiph. femur and tibia not fused with shaft)

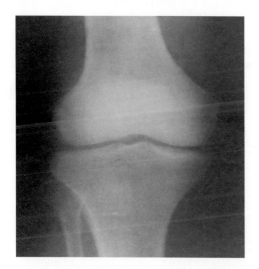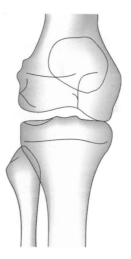

Fig. 9.6h: Age above 19 years (epiph. upper end fibula fused with shaft)

Sequence of Ossification and Union at the Ankle and Foot (Figs 9.7a to f)

Appearance

Present at birth

	– Calcaneum
	– Talus
6th month	– Cuboid (may be present at birth)
1st year	– Lower end of tibia
	– Lower end of fibula
	– Lateral cuneiform
2nd year	– Medial cuneiform
3rd year	– Intermediate cuneiform
	– Navicular
	– Base of first metatarsal
	– Heads of second, third, fourth and fifth metatarsals
	– Bases of phalanges
7th year	– Medial malleolus becomes bony
8th year	– Epiphysis for the posterior part of calcaneum

Fusion

16th year	– Fusion of epiphysis for the posterior part of calcaneum.
17th year	– Fusion of lower end of tibia with shaft.
	– Fusion of lower end of fibula with shaft.
18th year	– Fusion of the epiphyses of metatarsals and phalanges.

Fig. 9.7a: Ankle and foot—ossification and union

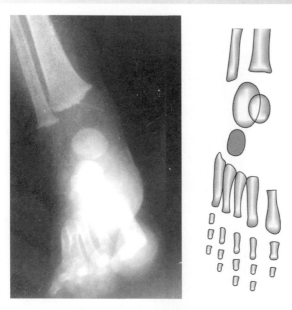

Fig. 9.7b: At birth (calcaneum and talus present)

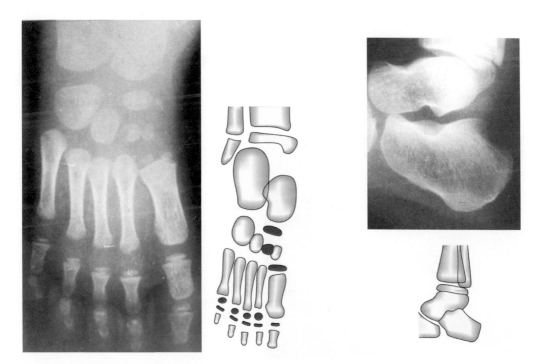

Fig. 9.7c: Age above 3 years (inter, cuneiform, navicular, epiph. base of 1st and heads of 2nd to 5th metatarsals present) and below 8 years (epiph. post, part calcaneum absent)

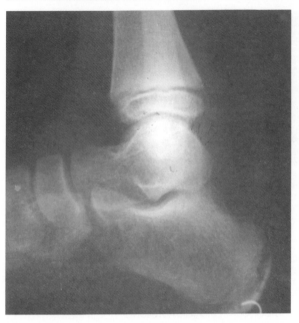
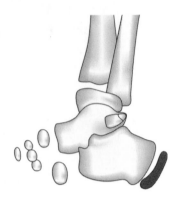

Fig. 9.7d: Age above 8 years (epiph. post part calcaneum present) below 16 years (epiph. calcaneum not fused to its body)

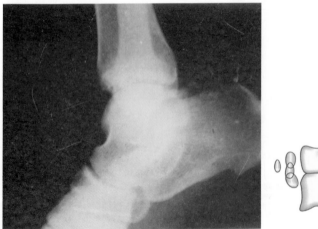
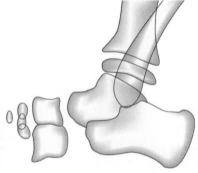

Fig. 9.7e: Age above 16 years (epiph. calcaneum fused with its body) below 17 years (epiph, lower end of tibia not fused with shaft)

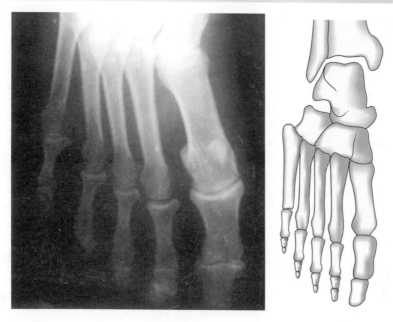

Fig. 9.7f: Age above 18 years (epiph of metatarsals fused with their shafts)

GENERALISATION

1. Bone age estimates the percentage of completed growth more accurately than chronological age. It is only occasionally helpful diagnostically but is valuable in predicting:
   a. final height
   b. age of reaching adult stature.
   c. puberty timing (when bone age is very discrepant from chronological age, e.g. a 9-year-old child with bone age of 6-year will probably enter puberty late compared to his peers.)
2. The ossification centres which are normally present at birth are in three long bones and three short bones. They may be recalled by the following mnemonic.

Full-Term Child Has These Centres

The initial letters refer to
- Femur (distal epiphysis)
- Tibia (proximal epiphysis)
- Calcaneum
- Humerus (proximal epiphysis)
- Talus
- Cuboid

Ossification of the distal end of femur occurs during the last two foetal months. Absence of the centre at birth is good presumptive evidence of prematurity and appearance is medicolegal evidence of full-term development.

3. In early childhood, the small bones of the foot undergo the most rapid changes and, therefore, are most satisfactory for evaluation of development in the early months Note that the first three tarsals (calcaneum, talus and cuboid) ossify in order of size.

4. After six months of age, the wrist and hands are more useful. Usually the carpal centres are not present at birth, but the first (capitate) appears at about two months of age. Note that the first three carpals (capitate, hamate and triquetral) ossify in order of size. Note also the spiral sequence of ossification in the carpus, starting with the largest and proceeding to the next largest in the same row, but omitting the pisiform capitate, hamate, triquetral, lunate, scaphoid, trapezium and trapezoid.

   All the metacarpal and phalangeal epiphyseal centres normally are demonstrable radiologically during the third year.

   The ossification of the distal radial epiphysis occurs at about 1 year of age.

   The distal ulnar epiphysis is present at 6 to 8 years of age in girls and at about 7 to 10 years of age in boys.

   In girls, the appearance of a sesamoid bone at the distal end of the first metacarpal indicates the menarche (age at which menses begin) within one or two years.

5. The postnatal ossification centres that have the highest statistical "communality" and hence the greatest predictive value in skeletal assessment are located in the hand, foot and knee. Thus three radiographs can actually provide more diagnostically useful in formation than the larger number often made. At puberty, however, more attention must be given to the centres of the hip, iliac bones, and the sesamoids of the thumb and other fingers.

6. As with other criteria of normal growth and development,normal variations must be taken into consideration. Thus there are racial and sex variations in bone maturation. Negroes show more rapid early maturation than Caucasians; skeletal development of girls is advanced over that of boys slightly so at birth but by as much as two years at puberty. In general osseous development correlates well with weight, height, and sexual development. Correlation of bone age with age at menarche is closer than that of chronological age and age at menarche.

Table 9.1: Chronological order of appearance of osseous centres

At birth	Ist year	2nd year	3rd year	4th year	5th year
Head of humerus		Greater tuberosity			Lesser tuberosity
	Capitulum and lateral part of trochlea				Head of radius
	Lower end of radius, capitate, hamate	Heads of 2nd-5th matacarpals bases proximal phalanges	Triquetral bases of first matacarpal, middle and terminal phalanges	Lunate	Scaphoid trapezium trapezoid
	Head of femur			Greater trochanter	
Lower end of femur upper end of tibia				Upper end of fibula	Patella
Cuboid	Lower end of tibia lower end of fibula lateral cuneiform	Medial cuneiform	Intermediate cuneiform navicular heads matatarsals first metatarsal base bases of phalanges		

Table 9.2: Chronological order of appearance of osseous centres

6th year	8th year	9th year	10th year	12th year
Fusion of the epiphysis upper end of humerus				
Medial epicondyle		Medial part of trochlea	Top of olecranon process	Lateral epicondyle
Lower end of ulna				Pisiform
	Fusion pubis with ischium			Lesser trochanter
			Tibial tubercle	
Bases of distal phalanges	Posterior part of calcaneum			

Table 9.3: Chronological order of appearance of union of epiphysis with diaphysis

15th year	16th year	17th year	18th year	19th year	20th year
					Fusion of upper end, of humerus with shaft
Olecranon	Lateral epicondyle, capitulum trochlea	Head of radius			Medial epicondyle
		Base of first metacarpal	Lower end of ulna radius metatarsals and bases phalanges	Lower end of radius	
	Lesser trochanter greater trochanter	Head of femur			Three parts of hip bone
			Lower end of femur upper end of tibia	Upper end of fibula	
	Posterior part of calcaneum	Lower end of tibia lower end of fibula	Epiphysis of metatarsals and phalanges		

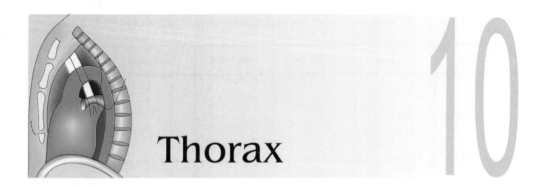

Thorax

10

CHEST

The importance of X-ray examination of the chest is very great in diseases of the lungs and heart. The ordinary standard X-ray film of chest is a postero-anterior view (PA) that is to say one taken with the film against the front of the patient's chest and the X-ray tube two metres behind the patient. With the subject sitting or standing the hands are placed on the waist and the elbows are pointed antero-laterally. This moves the scapulae from the lung fields. The skiagram is taken when the breathing is momentarily stopped after taking a deep inspiration.

RADIOGRAPHIC APPEARANCES

Postero-anterior View (Fig. 10.1)

● **Breasts** appear as homogenous opacities limited below by a crescentic margin. If the breasts are large and pendulous the shadow of this margin lies in the subdiaphragmatic area, while the lower parts of both lung fields show loss of translucency.

● **Cardiovascular shadow.** It is due to heart and great vessels and has a right and left border.

    a. **The right border** is venous and is formed from above downwards by:
- right innominate vein
- superior vena cava
- right atrium. It forms the right arc of cardiac shadow and extends from the base of the aorta as far as the diaphragm. When the heart is in the normal position, this arc moderately overlaps the vertebral shadows.
- inferior vena cava. It lies at the junction of the heart shadow with the diaphragm (cardiophrenic angle).

    b. **The left border** is formed from above downwards by:
- left subclavian artery
- arch of aorta (aortic knuckle)

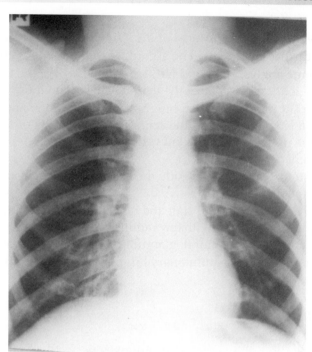

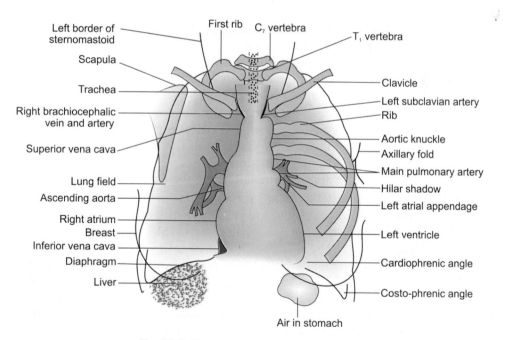

Left border of
sternomastoid

First rib   C₇ vertebra

T₁ vertebra

Scapula

Clavicle

Trachea

Left subclavian artery

Right brachiocephalic
vein and artery

Rib

Superior vena cava

Aortic knuckle

Axillary fold

Lung field

Main pulmonary artery

Ascending aorta

Hilar shadow

Right atrium

Left atrial appendage

Breast

Left ventricle

Inferior vena cava

Diaphragm

Cardiophrenic angle

Liver

Costo-phrenic angle

Air in stomach

Fig. 10.1: Thorax—postero-anterior view

- auricle of the left atrium
- left ventricle. It forms most of the left border of the cardiac shadow.
- The cardiac shadow will be according to the shape of the heart

● **Cardiophrenic angles,** right and left, are formed where the domes, covered by the diaphragmatic pleura, meet the lateral walls of the thorax.

● **Diaphragm:** The radiological diaphragm, convex upwards, consists of two domes, a right and a left, separated in the centre by the shadow of the heart (the right atrium on the right side and the left ventricle on the left side). The right dome is 2 to 4 cm higher than the left.

● **Fundus of stomach:** On the left side the air in the stomach stands out as a dark area below the diaphragm.

● **Hilar shadows:** In the normal state the hila appear as two thin paint-brush like shadows, quite distinct and with few ramifications. The images of the hila consist of vascular, bronchial and lymphoglandular components and of interstitial tissue. The neighbourhood of the pulmonary hilum is divided for descriptive purposes into:

  i. *Supra-hilar region*
  ii. *Peri-hilar region*
  iii. *Infra-hilar region*

An axial projection of a vessel (end on) gives perfectly circular opacity, which should not be mistaken for a pulmonary lymph node.

● **Lung fields:** The translucency of the lung parenchyma is due to the presence of air in the alveoli and bronchi. The fine mesh structure distinguishable on the X-ray film and which is commonly called, 'pulmonary stroma' is mainly due to a fine and rich system of arteries, veins and lymphatics. The peripheral ends of larger vascular units originate in the pulmonary hilar. For radiological purposes the lung fields are divided into three zones

  i. *Upper zone*—extends from the apex to a line drawn through the lower borders of the anterior ends of the second costal cartilages. The apex of each lung is seen to extend above the clavicles in this zone. Upper zone can be further sub-divided into the following regions.
    • Supraclavicular or apical—situated above the clavicles.
    • Infraclavicular—situated below the clavicles.
  ii. *Middle zone*—extends from the lower limit of upper zone to a line drawn through the lower borders of the fourth costal cartilages and contains the hila of the lungs.
  iii. *Lower zone (Basal)*—extends from lower limit of midzone to the base of the lungs.

Transparency of lung fields varies with each type of person. In fat people they are manifestly less transparent than in thin and wasted ones. In women the breasts diminish the transparency of lung fields. Usually the lung bases are clearer than the middle zone because of the thicker soft tissue on the chest wall in this region, and also because of the presence of the hilum and mediastinal ramifications.

- **Ribs:** The lungs are striped by the projection of the overlying ribs. Only the bony part of the ribs appear on radiographs. The costal cartilages do not show and so the anterior ends of ribs appear not to reach the sternum. The outline of the anterior portions of the ribs is clear than that of the posterior portions, because of the proximity to the film, but the posterior portions are more opaque because of their greater content of calcium salts. The anterior ends of the ribs are seen to lie at a lower level than the posterior ends. The posterior parts are directed downwards and laterally, the anterior parts downwards and medially.

  The posterior parts of the ribs behind the mediastinal shadow and below the level of the diaphragm are not seen.
- The first rib can be identified by noting the following characteristics.
  - Its broad anterior end.
  - Its articulation with the first thoracic vertebra (Tl) whose transverse process is inclined upwards and laterally in contrast to the transverse process of seventh cervical vertebra (C7) which has its transverse process directed downwards and laterally.

  Abnormalities of ribs concerning their number and shape are relatively common. Cervical ribs, unilateral or bilateral, give apical shadow.
- **Scapulae:** The medial borders and inferior angles of the scapulae are easily recognised. They mask some pulmonary details.
- **Sub-diaphragmatic area:** On the right side the radiopacity of liver shadow merges with the dome of the diaphragm.
- **Trachea:** Only its upper half is seen as transparent tube, with the lower cervical and upper thoracic vertebrae seen through it. It normally lies in the median plane but towards its bifurcation it usually inclines somewhat to the right.

Right or Left Lateral View (Fig. 10.2)

When right or left lateral view of the chest is desired that side of the person is placed closest to the film, and the arms are raised out of the projection as much as possible.
- **Cardiac shadow** rests on the anterior half of the diaphragm.
- **Cupolae of diaphragm** can be identified inferiorly by their different levels. The left is at higher level with the gastric air bubble just beneath its upper border, somewhat anterior to the mid line.
- **Descending aorta** can be identified in the retrocardiac space.
- **Inferior angles of the scapulae** are often seen superimposed on this regions.
- **Lung fields** extended posteriorly for about 1.5 cm behind the bodies of the thoracic vertebrae and inferiorly up to the diaphragm. The posteroinferior part of the lung which cannot be seen in an anterior view, since it lies below the level of the highest point of the dome of the diaphragm, can readly be examined in a lateral view. The upper part of the lung fields are somewhat obscured by the shoulder girdles.
- **Oesophagus** lies in the retrocardiac space anterior to the descending arorta. It can be seen only if it is filled with a contrast medium.
- **Retrosternal space** is the translucent space between the heart and the sternum.

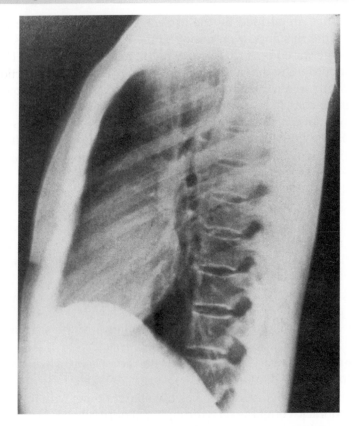

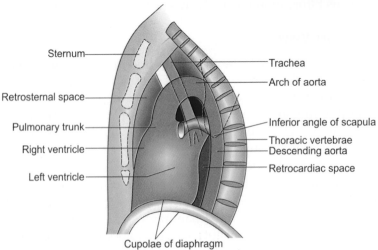

Sternum —

Trachea

Retrosternal space —

Arch of aorta

Pulmonary trunk —

Inferior angle of scapula

Right ventricle —

Thoracic vertebrae
Descending aorta

Left ventricle —

Retrocardiac space

Cupolae of diaphragm

Fig. 10.2: Thorax—lateral view

- **Retrocardiac space** is the translucent space separating the heart from the thoracic vertebrae.
- **Sternum** is seen anteriorly.
- **Thoracic vertebrae** are clearly seen posteriorly.
- **Trachea** appears as a translucent tube coming down from the neck up to the level of the sixth thoracic vertebra.

The Right Anterior Oblique View (Fig. 10.3)

In this position the patient is rotated so that his right side is in contact with the casette, and he is rotated away from the casette approximately 45°. This view is valuable for visualisation of oesophagus, the left atrium, the arch of the aorta and the mediastinal glands.

- **Arch of aorta** is fore-shortened and may be recognised curving posteriorly from the upper end of the heart shadow.
- **Ascending aorta** is seen arising from the upper end of the heart shadow. It is separated from the sternum by the translucent retrosternal space which actually is the anterior mediastinum and contains some lymph nodes.
- **Clavicle and sterno-clavicular joint of right side** are seen in the upper part of the skiagram.
- **Descending arota** is situated in the retrocardiac space just anterior to the bodies of the vertebrae.
- **Dome of the left side of the diaphragm** is seen in the lower part of the skiagram.
- **Heart shadow** is seen extending up from the anterior half of the dome of diaphragm. Anteriorly it lies close to the sternum and may overlap it.
- **Left atrium** (LA) and lower down the **Right atrium** (RA) are in contact with the oesophagus.
- **Lung fields**, right and left, are partly overlapped.
- **Prevertebral window** is a triangular translucent area between the vertebrae and the brachio-cephalic shadow.
- **Pulmonary trunk bifurcation and the left pulmonary veins** cast a round or oval shadow anterior to or partly overlapping the left bronchus.
- **Retrocardiac space** separates the heart from the spine posteriorly.
- **Descending aorta and oesophagus** lie in the retrocardiac space which represents the posterior mediastinum. Oesophagus is visible only when filled with a contrast medium.
- **Superior vascular pedicle or brachiocephalic shadow** formed by the brachiocephalic veins and the innominate, left common carotid and left subclavian arteries is seen extendin from the top of the arch of aorta.
- **Trachea** is seen as a dark tubular shadow, going downwards from the neck, crossing the shadow of the arch of aorta and then dividing into right and left bronchus about 3.75 cm anterior to the body of the sixth thoracic vertebra.

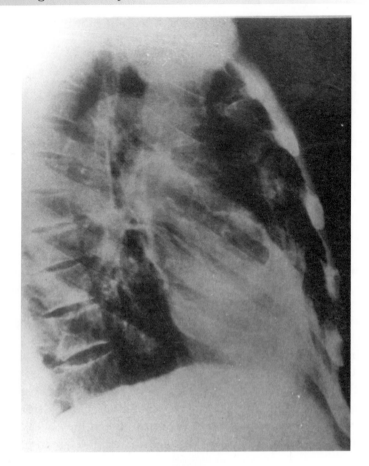

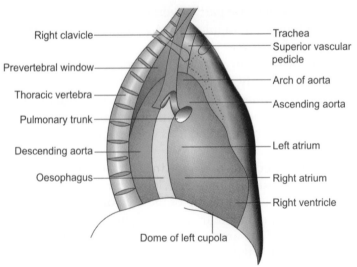

Fig. 10.3: Thorax—right anterior-oblique view

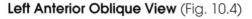

Left Anterior Oblique View (Fig. 10.4)

In this position the subject is rotated 45° with the left shoulder anterior against the cassette.

- **Aortic arch** is seen in its entirety. It takes a rather wide sweep so that the upper part of the descending aorta overlaps the vertebral bodies posteriorly.
- **Aortic triangle** is a translucent triangular area in the upper part of the skiagram. It is bounded below by the top of the aortic arch, anteriorly by the superior vascular pedicle (the edge is formed by the oesophagus and left subclavian artery) and posteriorly by the thoracic vertebrae.
- **Aortic window** is a translucent space bounded above by the aortic arch, below by the left atrium, to the right by the descending aorta and to the left by the ascending aorta and the pulmonary trunk.
- **Clavicle (of left side)** is conspicuous.
- **Cupola (Lt) of the diaphragm** appears to the right of the skiagram.
- **Heart shadow** has the left ventricle just in front of the anterior margin of the thoracic spine. This is the posterior basilar portion of the left ventricle (LV). Above this lies the left atrium (LA). The anterior margin of the silhouette is formed inferiorly by the right ventricle (RV) and above this by the right atrium (RA). This is the only view in which the right ventricle is adequately and definitely seen.
- **Pulmonary artery of left side** is seen in the clear space above the left atrium.
- **Trachea** passes downwards across the aortic window as a translucent tube.

BRONCHOGRAPHY

It is used to visualise the bronchial tree and is an important aid for diagnosis and localisation of lung diseases.

Method for Bronchography

Dionosil aqueous (an iodine preparation) is used as a contrast medium.

A. Pre-bronchographic preparation

- The patient is treated with an antibiotic for a few days to clear any infection out of the bronchial tree.
- Respiratory efficacy is assessed by clinical examination on the day of bronchography.
- Nothing is given orally.
- A sedative is administered to allay anxiety.
- Atropine 1/100 gr. is given by intramuscular injection 45 minutes before bronchography to decrease secretions and thus avoid the dilution of the dye with respiratory secretions.
- Sensitivity test to the local dye is done by injecting 0.1 cc of dye intracutaneously.

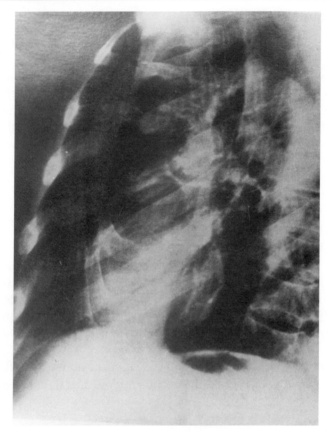

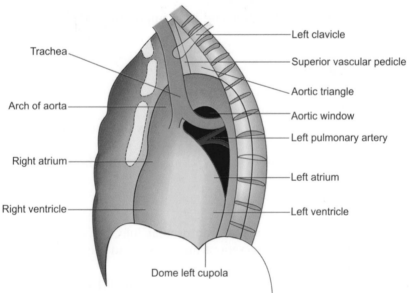

Trachea

Arch of aorta

Right atrium

Right ventricle

Left clavicle

Superior vascular pedicle

Aortic triangle

Aortic window

Left pulmonary artery

Left atrium

Left ventricle

Dome left cupola

Fig. 10.4: Thorax—left anterior-oblique view

B. Technique of bronchography

- The procedure is explained to the patient to gain his confidence.
- The throat is sprayed with 2 per cent local anaesthetic at intervals of 5 to 7 mts. Usually 3 to 4 sprays are sufficient to anaesthetise the throat and this is confirmed by testing for the absence of pharyngeal and palatal reflexes, at the same time the patient also complains of difficulty in swallowing.
- The anaesthetic is sprayed over the posterior pharyngeal wall, palate, pillars, fossae, posterior part of the tongue, epiglottis and deep over the carina. During the spray the tongue should be pulled out with the help of a piece of gauze to get a good field. After this endotracheal injection of local anaesthetic is given through the cricothyroid membrane. As an alternative it can be injected from the back of tongue with the help of a laryngeal cannula. Usually it takes about 6 to 7 ml of local anaesthetic to anaesthetise both sides of the bronchial tree and trachea.
    i. *Endotracheal catheterisation:* In this procedure the dye is put in with the help of a catheter passed through the nose into the trachea.
    Usually 10 cc of dye is required for opacifying one side of bronchial tree.
    ii. *Bronchoscopic route:* This is very much similar to the endotracheal catheterisation except that the bronchoscope is used in place of a catheter and the dye is injected through it.

After injecting the dye by any of the above procedures the patient is subjected to screening and chest skiagrams are taken in the following positions.

(a) For unilateral purpose
- PA
- Lateral views.

(b) For bilateral purposes
- PA
- Right anterior oblique and left anterior oblique views.

(C) Post-bronchographic period

- After bronchography the patient is not allowed to take anything orally for two hours as there could be a danger of aspiration.
- Postural drainage is resorted to help early elimination of the dye from the lungs.

Anterior Bronchogram (Fig. 10.5)

The various segmental bronchi can be recognised as under:

Right Lung

(a) **Upper lobe bronchus** arises postero-superiorly a short distance from the trachea and is a short and wide air tube directed laterally. It divides into its three segmental branches.
    i. *Apical bronchus* passes upwards towards the medial third of the clavicle.
    ii. *Anterior bronchus* directed downwards and laterally.

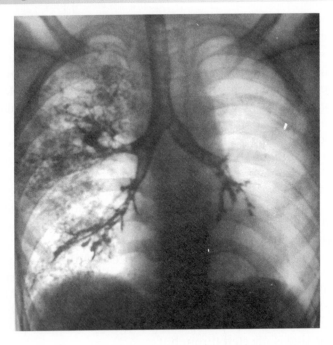

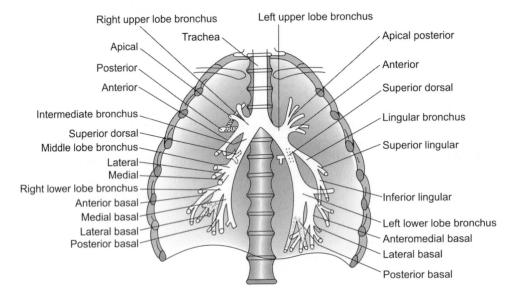

Fig. 10.5: Anterior view of bronchial tree

iii. *Posterior bronchus* lies mostly posterior to apical bronchus and so is not clearly distinguishable. The continuation of the main trunk is called the intermediate bronchus.

b. **Middle lobe bronchus** arises anteromedially from the intermediate bronchus and divides into two segmental branches for the supply of the middle lobe.
   i. *Medial and*
   ii. *Lateral*

These segmental bronchi overlap the lateral basal bronchus of the lower lobe.

c. **Lower lobe bronchus**
   i. *Superior or dorsal bronchus* arises posterolaterally from the intermediate bronchus and is directed backwards. It is seen as a ring shadow with small radiating branches near the level of origin of middle lobe bronchus opposite 7th thoracic vertebra.
   The further continuation of the main bronchial trunk is the basal bronchus which subdivides to form four basal segmental bronchi.
   ii. *Lateral basal bronchus* overlapped by middle lobe bronchi.
   iii. *Medial basal*
   iv. *Anterior basal* and
   v. *Posterior basal bronchi*—cast their shadows close together more medial to the one by lateral lobe bronchus.

Left Lung

The left main bronchus is considerably longer than the right.

a. **Left upper lobe bronchus** is seen at a lower level than the right one. It arises anterosuperiorly from the main bronchus and divides into two divisions. The upper division usually subdivides into two segmental bronchi.
   i. *Apical posterior bronchus* is directed upwards towards the medial third of the clavicle.
   ii. *Anterior bronchus* is directed upwards and laterally.
   Lingular bronchus gives the following segmental bronchi.
   i. *Superior lingular and*
   ii. *Inferior lingular bronchi* which are directed downwards and laterally

b. **Lower lobe bronchus** is short given after a few millimetres.
   i. *Superior segmental (dorsal) bronchus* is immediately below the level of origin of the upper lobe bronchus. The lower lobe bronchus then continues as the basal bronchus which subdivides to form the basal segmental bronchi.
   ii. *Lateral basal bronchus* is just below the lingular bronchus.
   iii. *Anteromedial.* The small medial and somewhat larger anterior basal bronchi arise from a common stem, and is called the anteromedial basal bronchus.
   iv. *Posterior basal* which along with the anteromedial basal bronchus is placed more medially.

LATERAL BRONCHOGRAMS

Right Lung (Fig. 10.6)

● **Upper lobe bronchus** is seen end on at the intervertebral disc between D5 and D6 vertebrae. Its three segmental bronchi are seen as follows.
  i. *Apical bronchus* is directed up.
  ii. *Anterior bronchus* is directed downwards and forwards.
  iii. *Posterior bronchus* goes upwards and backwards.
● **Middle lobe bronchus**
  i. *Lateral* and
  ii. *Medial bronchi* are directed forwards parallel to the anterior bronchus and a little below it.

Lower Lobe Bronchus

  i. *Superior (dorsal) bronchus* is directed backwards at about the same level (D7) as the middle lobe bronchus.
  ii. *Posterior basal bronchus* overlaps the vertebral column and is directed into the constodiaphragmatic angle.
  iii. *Anterior basal bronchus* is seen overlapping the shadows of diaphragm and liver.
  iv. *Lateral basal and*
  v. *Medial basal bronchi* appear between the anterior and posterior basal bronchi.

Left Lung (Fig. 10.7)

Upper lobe bronchus

  i. *Apical posterior bronchus* has radiating branches directed upwards into the apex and the region behind it.
  ii. *Anterior bronchus* goes upwards and forwards.

Lingular Bronchus

  i. *Superior* and
  ii. *Inferior lingular bronchi* are seen directed downwards and forwards at the level of the intervertebral disc between D6 and D7 vertebrae.

Lower lobe bronchus

  i. *Superior (dorsal) bronchus* passes backward opposite D7 vertebra.
  ii. *Lateral* and
  iii. *Posterior basal bronchi* can be recognised as on the right side, mainly between the heart shadow and vertebral column.

Oesophageogram (Fig. 10.8)

Barium swallow is the standard method of examination of the oesophagus.

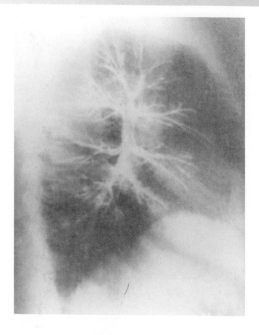

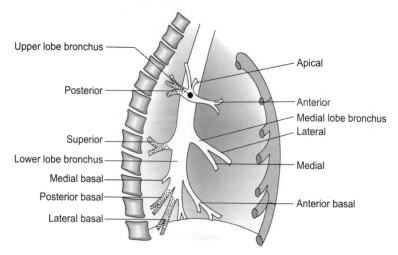

Upper lobe bronchus

Posterior

Superior

Lower lobe bronchus

Medial basal

Posterior basal

Lateral basal

Apical

Anterior

Medial lobe bronchus

Lateral

Medial

Anterior basal

Fig. 10.6: Right bronchogram in lateral view

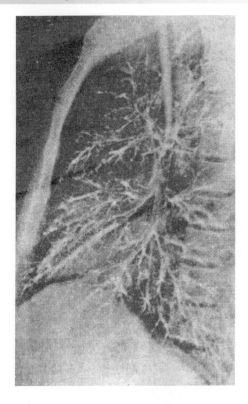

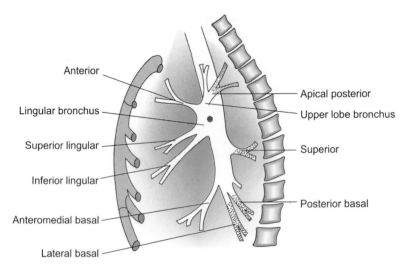

Fig. 10.7: Left bronchogram in lateral view

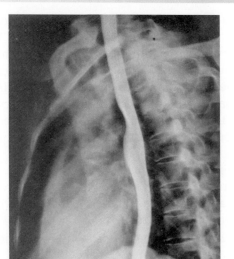

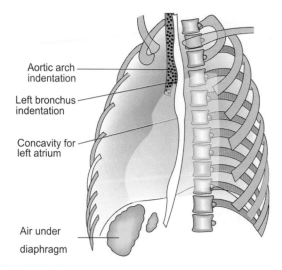

Aortic arch indentation

Left bronchus indentation

Concavity for left atrium

Air under diaphragm

Fig. 10.8: Oesophageogram—left anterior-oblique view

The material used is barium sulphate mixed with water to form a 50% suspension.

Oesophageograms are radiographs of the chest, with barium delineating the oesophagus, obtained in posterio-anterior, oblique and lateral projections.

The proper examination involves a combination of fluoroscopy and radiography. The patient stands behind the fluoroscopic screen and is asked to take several swallows of the thin barium mixture. This is watched as it passes through the entire oesophagus and into the stomach and the patient is rotated into various positions so that the entire circumference of the oesophagus is brought into profile. X-ray films are taken during the fluoroscopic study.

A left anterior oblique view for example will show three shallow concave indentation on the barium shadow. From above downwards they are

1. First is due to the aortic arch and immediately below this there is frequently a second shallower indentation due to.
2. The left bronchus. Lower down a long shallower anterior concavity due to
3. The left atrium.

We depend upon the oesophagus to delineate most accurately the retrocardiac structures, as it is a close anterior relation of descending aorta. In view of these relations enlargements of the atria or descending thoracic aorta can be diagnosed by observing the oesophageal displacements caused by them.

Abdomen and Pelvis

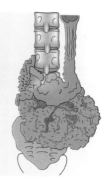

PLAIN X-RAY ABDOMEN

A plain rediograph of the abdomen is extremely valuable in
  i. Excluding biliary and renal calculi,
  ii. In urgent surgery for diagnosing:
     • acute intestinal obstruction.
     • paralytic ileus and
     • rupture of a hollow viscus.

It is taken after preparing the patient in the following manner to eliminate excessive faecal, air and gas shadows from the intestine.
   • Purgative should be given 36 or 24 hours before X-ray is taken. Half to one ounce of castor oil is effective in clearing the colon with most patients, but it tends to encourage gas distension after the initial irritation. Milder purgatives such as Senna may also be used. Colon wash-outs may also be given.
   • Patient should be up and about before examination to dispel gases when this is possible.
   • Pitressin (1.5 ml) can also be given subcutaneously to cause the colon to empty, provided the patient is not pregnant or suffering from high blood pressure. After the injection the patient is instructed to retire to the lavatory and pass flatus. The radiographs are then taken.

RADIOGRAPHIC APPEARANCE

Antero-posterior View (Fig. 11.1)

This X-ray of the abdomen is also called "KUB" film, since it is usually employed in the examination of the urinary tract and the letters symbolise "Kidneys, Ureters and Bladder". The following features are noticeable.
a. **Bony structures**
   • Coccyx
   • Iliac crests

153

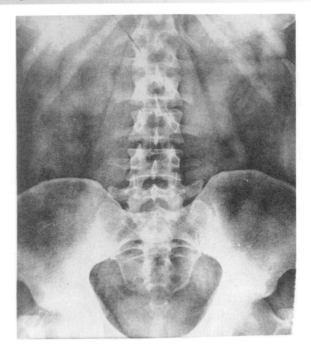

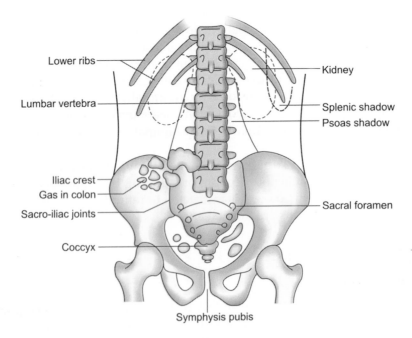

Lower ribs

Kidney

Lumbar vertebra

Splenic shadow
Psoas shadow

Iliac crest
Gas in colon
Sacro-iliac joints

Sacral foramen

Coccyx

Symphysis pubis

Fig. 11.1: Abdomen—plain X-ray (KUB)

- Lower ribs
- Lumbar vertebrae
- Sacral foramina
- Sacro-iliac joints
- Symphysis pubis

b. **Soft tissues**
   - **Alimentary canal:** It shows dark areas of translucency due to contained gas e.g. the air in the fundus of stomach and splenic flexure of large bowel can be seen below the left dome of diaphragm.
   - **Kidneys:** Cast clear shadow on each side of vertebral column.
   - **Liver** casts a shadow which merges with the right dome of the diaphragm above and sometimes presents a well defined lower border close to the right costal margin. In the middle line the shadow merges with that of the heart and vertebrae, and the left extremity of the shadow of the liver is superimposed on the transparent gas bubble of the stomach and is usually not recognisable.
   - **Psoas muscle:** It can be clearly seen with a well defined lateral margin extending downwards and outwards.
   - **Spleen:** Its lateral part can often be identified on the left side.

CONTRAST RADIOGRAPHY

GASTROINTESTINAL TRACT

The alimentary tract is examined with the aid of a contrast medium. Their common value depends on their outlining the internal shape of hollow organs. The most commonly employed medium in present day radiography of the gastrointestinal tract is barium sulphate in water suspension. 125 gm of barium sulfate powder to 180 ml of water is adequate in most patients. If the small intestines are to be examined an additional 120 to 180 ml of the mixture should be given routinely.

BARIUM MEAL

Barium meal is flavoured with vanilla and sweetend with white saccharin. It has a creamy consistency. Before giving barium meal the patient is prepared in the following manner.
- He should have nothing to eat or drink for six hours prior to the barium meal and should not smoke, chew gum or take medicines during this period.
- No purgative should be given the night before the examination as they tend to cause misleading motor phenomena.
- Medicines containing elements of high atomic weight such as bismuth, calcium or magnesium should be discontinued at least three days prior to the test as they may adhere to colon wall in the region of splenic flexure and cast a confusing shadow.

The meal is best given at about 9 am. The patient drinks 0.5 to 1 pint (10 to 15 oz) of barium emulsion so that stomach is filled up. The barium emulsion is then smeared over the interior of the stomach by gentle pressure on the abdominal wall. The patient is radiographed immediately after the meal and then at 1/2 hr, 1 hr and 1½ hours intervals. The stomach starts emptying its contents within a few minutes of their reaching it. A half pint of barium suspension will usually have left the stomach in two hours.

RADIOGRAPHIC APPEARANCE

(A) Stomach (Figs 11.2a to e)

In most subjects in the standing position the stomach is 'J' shaped or Fish hook' type. 'Steer-horn' type of stomach runs obliquely downwards and to the right and narrows towards the pyloric end.

- **Position of stomach** is subject to wide variations. It is assessed by reference to incisura angularis. The stomach is higher in broad and stoky type of individuals than in the slender type. It is fixed at its cardiac end just to the left of the eleventh thoracic vertebral body, and by the first part of duodenum to the posterior abdominal wall just to the right of the second lumbar vertebra. Between these points it can vary in position according to its degree of distension and the posture of the patient. The only guides to its location are that in the recumbent person it rarely extends below the level of the anterior-superior iliac spines and that greater part of it lies to the left of the midline.
- **Fundus:** The translucent gas bubble (German-magenblase) outlines the fundus.
- **Greater curvature:** Outlines the gas bubble and then runs more or less parallel to the lesser curvature but usually shows a bulge opposite the incisura angularis. This curvature is more irregular in outline, especially in the descending part, on account of indentations caused by the irregularly disposed gastric rugae. It forms an acute permanent angle the cardiac notch, with the left border of the oesophagus. Notches due to peristaltic wave may be seen in the distal half of the greater curvature.
- **Incisura angularis:** At the junction of the body with the pyloric antrum the lesser curvature increase abruptly to form this angular notch.
- **Lesser curvature:** It runs almost vertically downwards to incisura angularis whence it passes upwards and to the right. It forms the right border of the stomach.
- **Pyloric antrum** is the wide part of the pyloric region narrowing to pyloric canal, the terminal part of which is surrounded by the pyloric sphincter.
- **Pyloric canal:** It appears as a column of barium, with parallel walls, about 2 to 3 mm wide and 5 to 8 mm long joining the pyloric antrum.

(B) Duodenum (Figs 11.2a to e)

The duodenum receives the barium meal intermittently from the stomach. Its four parts will be seen to have the following features.

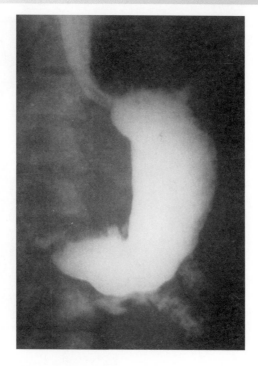

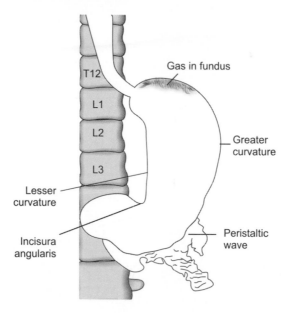

Fig. 11.2a: Stomach (J-shaped) immediately after barium meal

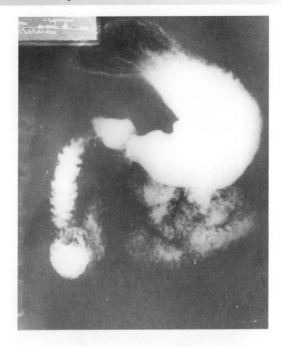

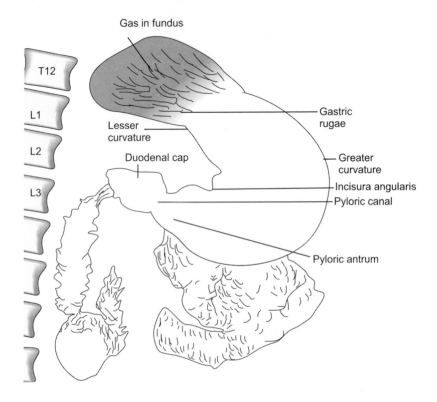

Fig. 11.2b: Stomach and duodenum—15 minutes after barium meal

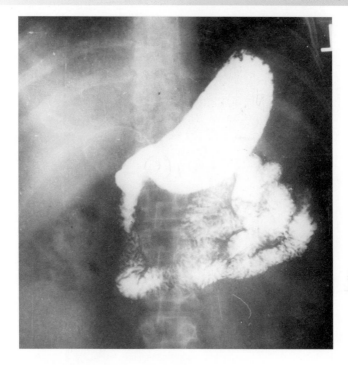

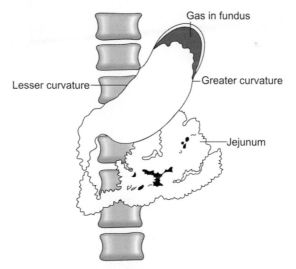

Fig. 11.2c: Stomach (Steer-horn) after barium meal

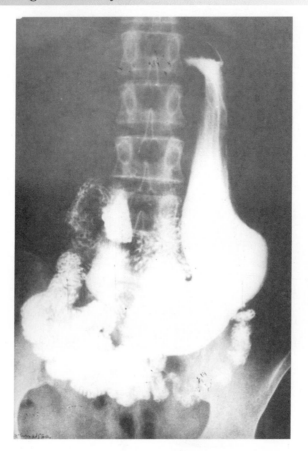

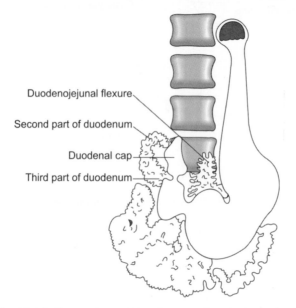

Duodenojejunal flexure

Second part of duodenum

Duodenal cap

Third part of duodenum

Fig. 11.2d: Stomach and duodenum—30 minutes after barium meal

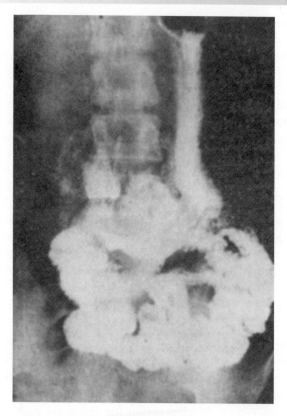

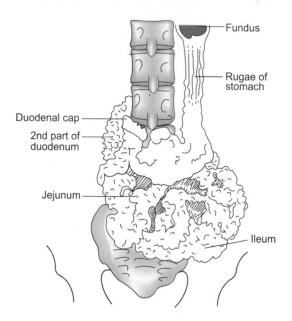

Fig. 11.2e: Stomach and small intestine 1½ hour after barium meal

● **First part (duodenal cap):** It functions as a separate entity. Its walls are smooth in outline and owing to the protrusion of the pyloric end into the lumen of this part of duodenum and its fixation to the abdominal wall, the opaque mass which temporarily fills it, assumes the form of a solid Nace of spades', triangular in shape with the base opposite the pyloric canal. The base forming a stem and leaf relationship with the pyloric canal. Usually it is upright, sometimes it lies on its side, sometimes it is directed sagittally. This part is known radiographically as the **duodenal cap**. Not only it is seen as an opaque mass but it lends itself particularly well to compression whereby the barium in it is thinned by pressure so that irregularities of the mucous membrane appear in relief. It most often shows signs of disease. Radiologically a "fleck" (from the German meaning "spot") is a loculation of barium of any size from a few millimetres to 2 or more centimetres which strongly suggests a break in the normal mucosal structure and ulceration. In view of the great frequency of ulceration in this area, the detection of a fleck in this location is of extreme importance.

● **Second part:** It gives a floccular shadow because the barium emulsion is broken up into small portions.

● **Third part:** It is seen running transversely.

● **Fourth part:** It is directed upwards and to the left.

● **Duodeno-jejunal flexure:** It is hidden behind the stomach shadow and is commonly seen above the incisura angularis close to the lesser curvature.

The passage of barium through the second, third and fourth parts is rapid. There may be a short delay at the beginning of the third part.

The duodenum is in a fixed position for the most part, and hence variations from its normal position become of significance in the detection of space occupying lesions in adjoining structures, such as pancreas, lesser omental bursa, colon, gallbladder and biliary ducts. There is, however, a considerable variation in different individuals in the normal contour of the duodenum and this must be borne in mind when radiography of the duodenum is attempted.

(c) Jejunum and Ileum (Fig. 11.3)

Once the stomach, duodenum and upper coils of small intestine have been radiographed, X-ray films at half an hour, one hour and then at hourly intervals up to four hours until the caecum is filled, may suffice. If after the first hour the patient has a good barium meal again, filling of the distal small intestine will be much faster. Alternatively as soon as gastric emptying is well established, the patient is given 0.5 mg neostigmine subcutaneously. With this stimulus the whole small intestine and the proximal colon are usually well outlined within two hours, and the examination is thus speeded up without apparently any loss of diagnostic accuracy.

● **Proximal part of small intestine:** The barium shadow remains broken up and shows feather like appearance.

● **Middle part of the small intestine:** It lies somewhat to the left.

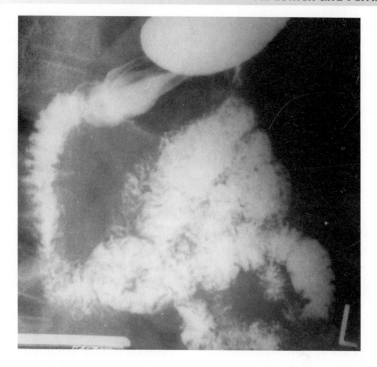

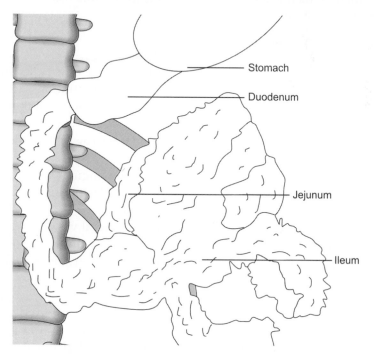

Fig. 11.3: Jejunum and ileum after barium meal

● **Distal part of ileurn:** It forms a more homogeneous shadow, coils are seen lying in the pelvis. Last few inches are narrower than the rest. The terminal part is seen running upwards and to the right to join the caecum on its inner side a short distance above its base.

Barium Enema

The large intestine can be examined after either a barium enema or a barium meal. A barium enema is used in preference for most purposes. A necessary preliminary is to cleanse the bowel thoroughly, and for this purpose the following procedure is adopted.
- A suitable purgative (castor oil 1–2 oz or Dulcolax tablets) is given 48 hours before the examination to remove gross faecal masses.
- A clear liquid diet is given for a period of 24 hours prior to X-ray.
- A high colonic wash-out is given just prior to the examination. Three pints of plain water or normal saline are run into the rectum from douche can, at a pressure of about one foot of water. No soap should be used for colonic lavage.

After the patient has been thus prepared the whole colon is easily outlined by slowly running in two to three pints of a simple barium sulphate suspension through the anus. 300 gm of barium sulfate powder are added to each 1000 ml of tap-water. Various drugs are sometimes added, e.g. Clysotrast to help colonic peristalsis and precipitate mucus which might otherwise cling to the mucosa. The result is an improved post evacuation study.

(D) Large Bowel (Fig. 11.4)

● **Appendix** may sometimes be seen arising from the base of the caecum.
● **Caecum and ascending colon:** Sacculations known as frustrations, are present in proximal part of colon but may not be evident in the distal part if the pressure is high.
● **Descending and pelvic colon:** Descending colon is narrower than the ascending portion. Pelvic colon may show a wide loop.
● **Hepatic and splenic flexures:** Owing to the acute angular curvatures in the regions of the colic flexures and pelvic colon, there is superimposition of loops in these regions.
● **Rectum** can be seen closely related to sacrum in a lateral view.
● **Transverse colon:** Particularly varies in length from quite a short one to a redundant loop. The normal large bowel shows many variations in form.

Biliary Tract

Visualisation of gallbladder requires a contrast medium to be introduced into it. Administration of an iodine compound which is excreted by the liver and is concentrated in the gallbladder renders the gallbladder radiopaque (Graham-Cole test). This method of visualisation of gallbladder is known as cholecystography.
  i. **Oral cholecystography:** Telepaque (iopanoic acid) containing 66% iodine by weight is the oral preparation of choice. It should not be given to patients

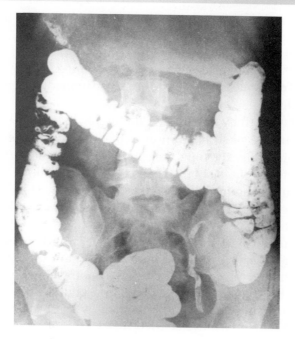

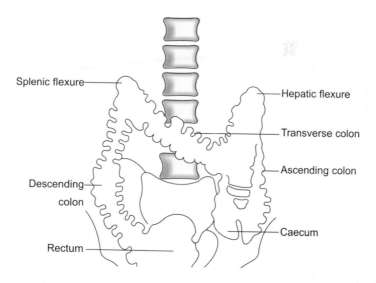

Splenic flexure

Hepatic flexure

Transverse colon

Ascending colon

Descending colon

Caecum

Rectum

Fig. 11.4: Large bowel after barium enema

suffering from uraemia, nephritis or diarrhoea. Another drug which has been introduced recently is Oragrafin (Sodium ipodate).

The patient is prepared in the following manner.

- A fat free evening meal is given at about 6 pm.
- Twelve Telepaque tablets (4 gm) are given immediately after the meal (Single oral method).
- Nothing is given by mouth after midnight.
- Film should be taken 14 hours after the ingestion of the tablets.
- Immediately after the films are exposed the patient is given a fatty meal (50 gm of butter, 2 slices of bread and one glass of milk)
- In an hour's time further radiographs are taken. These show the emptying capacity of the gallbladder and often reveal stones which may only become evident in the partially evacuated viscus.

ii. **Intravenous cholecystography:** It may be used for visualisation of the gallbladder if diarrhoea, pyloric obstruction or any other factor interferes with the absorption of the orally administered contrast medium. As there is risk of damage to the arm if the contrast medium should leak out of the vein during an intravenous injection, the oral method, which is nearly as reliable as the intravenous, should always be tried first.

Biligrafin (20% solution of sodium iodipamide) which contains 64% iodine is the preparation of choice. The drug must not be administered to a patient with hyperthyroidism or to one known to be sensitive to iodine. Sensitivity to iodine must be tested before administration.

- No preparation is required. Moderate exercise is the best means of dispelling gas from the intestine.
- One or two 20 ml ampoules are warmed and given intravenously slowly over a period of ten minutes.
- Serial films are taken 10, 20 or 30 minutes after injection to visualise the common bile duct.
- Film to demonstrate gallbladder should not be made until 1½ to 2 hours after injection as the gallbladder fills a considerable time after the ducts.
- If the gallbladder is visualised the usual fatty meal is given and further exposures are made after 30 minutes to demonstrate its power of contraction.
- When cholecystography is completely negative further films after five hours may demonstrate the biliary system.

RADIOGRAPHIC APPEARANCE

Cholecystogram (Figs 11.5a to c)

Note the following features of gallbladder in a cholecystogram.

- **Position:** It is usually seen in the angle between the twelfth rib and the upper lumbar vertebrae. The position is subject to considerable variation in normal subjects. It may occupy any part of quadrilateral whose vertical extent is from the upper border of the twelfth thoracic vertebra to the lower border of the fourth

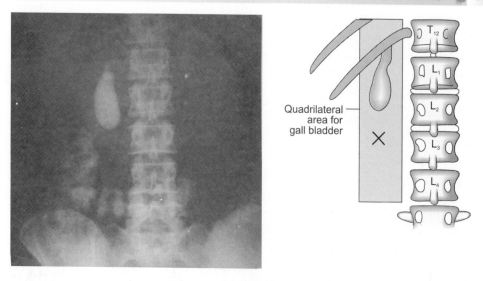

Fig. 11.5a: Gallbladder—position

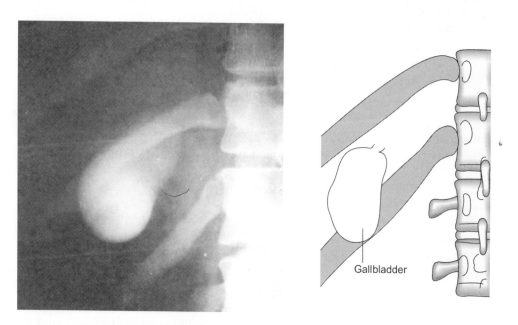

Fig. 11.5b: Gallbladder—cholecystogram before fatty meal

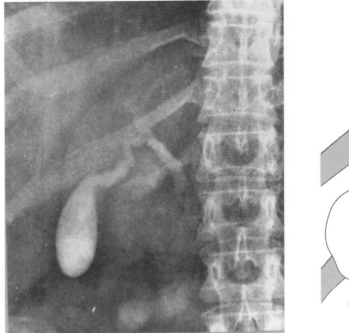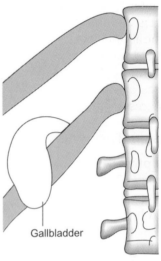

Gallbladder

Fig. 11.5c: Gallbladder—cholecystogram after fatty meal

lumbar vertebra and the transverse extent from a point 2.5 cm to the right of the median plane to a point 10 cm to the right of the median plane.

● **Shape and size:** Gallbladder appears as a pear-shaped homogeneous opacity. The density of the shadow is subject to considerable variation in normal individuals.

When the gallbladder is not visualised it may mean any one or more of the following possibilities*

- Markedly impaired liver function so that bile formation is impeded and the dye is not excreted.
- Obstructive disease of extra-hepatic bile ducts so that the dye does not reach the gallbladder.
- Pyloric obstruction or diarrhoea causing non-absorption of the dye.
- Diseased gallbladder (chronic cholecystitis) results in non-concentration of the dye. Non-function and occlusion of the gallbladder is demonstrated by the fact that the dye, although present in the bowel, is not seen in the gallbladder.

Subnormal function and the presence of non-opaque gall stones can also be demonstrated by the lack of the usual density of the shadow of the dye in the gallbladder in the former case, and by the presence of translucent shadows in the outline of the gallbladder in the latter case.

Urinary Tract

In a plain skiagram of abdomen (KUB film) the kidney outlines can be cleary seen. To outline the calyces, ureter and bladder, certain organic compounds containing iodine in their molecule, have to be introduced either intravenously or through a catheter to make the urinary tract radiopaque such an X-ray in which the urinary tract is visualised by a radiopaque medium is called a pyelogram. Plain radiographs of the abdomen should be taken first, before pyelography, as these will show whether the kidneys are normal in size, shape and position, and whether there are any abnormal opacities in the renal tract, which may require localisation by pyelography. Occasionally, they may reveal non-renal conditions which make pyelography unnecessary.

Descending Pyelogram

The preparation and technique is as follows:
Conray 420 (compound containing iodine) is the preparation of choice.
- A mild vegetable aperient on two consecutive evenings preceding examination.
- A light supper on the preceding evening.
- For twelve hours before the injection the intake of fluids is limited and diuretic drugs are excluded.
- No food or fluid is given on the morning of the test.
- Urinary bladder should be empty when the injection is given.
- If possible the patient should be up and about to expel gases.
- Test for iodine sensitivity is done.
- Warm 20–40 ml of the solution to body temperature. Inject slowly taking care that there is no leakage out of the vein.

The first radiograph of the abdomen is taken five minutes after the injection. A second radiograph ten minuts after the injection may suffice but more may be taken if considered necessary.

Excretion urography or descending or intravenous pyelography (IVP) is not only performed to obtain an anatomic evaluation of the urinary tracts, but is also done to determine the functional status of the kidneys and so constitutes one of the renal function tests.

RADIOGRAPHIC APPEARANCE

Descending Pyelogram (Fig. 11.6)

- **The bladder:** As time passes the amount of the contrast medium in the bladder increases so that its outline and position are easily shown.
- **The calyces:** Three major calyces will usually be recognised directed laterally. They are upper, middle and lower. The number may vary. Six to twelve cup-shaped minor calyces are situated at the end of the major calyces.
  A minor calyx consists of a neck and an expanded extremity cupped by projection of the renal pyramid into its lumen.

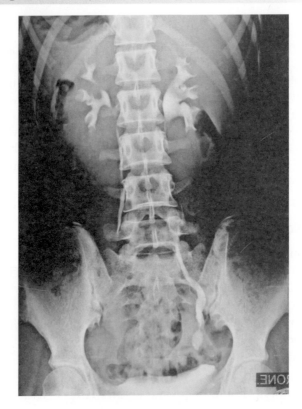

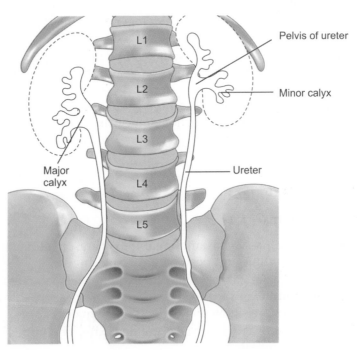

Fig. 11.6: Descending pyelogram

- **Kidney:** Generally the passage of the drug through the kidney is too fast to reach a useful concentration. If the outflow of secretion from the pelvis is prevented or if the kidney is flooded with a very large amount of the drug, the renal tissue becomes somewhat opaque to X-ray and a shadow of the kidney can be obtained (Nephrogram). Attempts have been made to use this effect to show disease process.
- **The pelvis of ureter** is funnel-shaped and narows towards it medial inferior angle. It joins the ureter at an obtuse angle. The upper border is somewhat convex and the inferior border presents a semi-circular concavity.
- **The ureters** run downwards close to tips of the transverse processes of the lumbar vertebrae, and in front of the sacro-iliac joints. In the pelvis they cast a shadow 1 cm on the medial side of the brim and across the tip of the ischical spine from where they turn medially to join the bladder shadow.

Ascending Pyelogram

If delineation of the calyces, pelves or ureters is unsatisfactory on one or both sides after intravenous pyelography, a retrograde pyelogram may be necessary. An intravenous pyelogram is safe, but a retrograde pyelogram must be undertaken with caution. The preparation and technique is as follows:

- Nothing by mouth after a light meal in the evening.
- Cleansing enema in the morning.
- A cystoscope is passed through the urethra into the bladder. A cystoscope is an instrument of such a size that it can be passed up the urethra. The inner end carries a small electric light and a mirror, the outer end a telescope, a system of lenses focused on the mirror. The light from the lamp luminates a part of the bladder wall. Its image is reflected by the minor along the tube into the eyepiece. Special channels are incorporated in the instrument through which fine flexible catheters can be passed and guided into the orifices and then up the ureters.
- A ureteric catheter is manipulated through the cystoscope into the bladder then under direct vision is guided into the ureter.
- Hypaque (45 per cent) is injected by the catheter into the ureter in a fully conscious patient.
- The injection of the opaque medium is continued until the patient feels discomfort in the loin, or until 10 ml have been introduced.
- The radiograph is taken.
- The fluid is aspirated from the renal pelvis and the catheter is removed.

RADIOGRAPHIC APPEARANCE

Ascending Pyelogram (Fig. 11.7)

The anatomic details are more satisfactory in a retrograde pyelograph than in an excretion pyelograph. The following can easily be visualised.

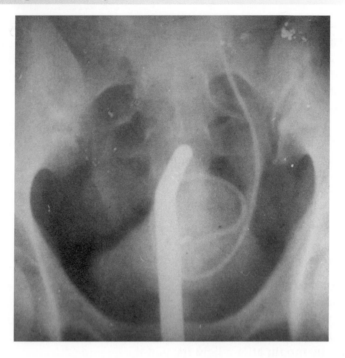

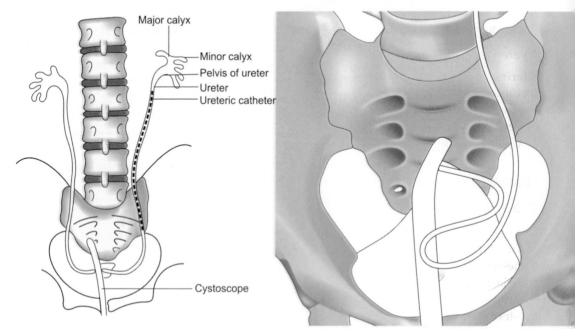

Major calyx

Minor calyx
Pelvis of ureter
Ureter
Ureteric catheter

Cystoscope

Fig. 11.7: Ascending pyelogram

- Cystoscope can be seen in the urinary bladder
- Major calyces
- Minor calyces
- Pelvis of the ureter
- Ureter
- Ureteric catheter is visible lying in the lumen of the ureter.

 ## FEMALE GENITAL TRACT

HYSTEROSALPINGOGRAPHY

It is particularly useful in cases of sterility and to prove or disprove the patency of the uterine tubes. It also outlines the uterine cavity, shows the length, shape and position of the fallopian tubes. The most common contrast medium used is Lipiodol. A suitable cannula, which at the same time obstructs the cervical canal, is inserted into the cervical canal of the uterus. Approximately 6 ml of the opaque medium is injected and an antero-posterior film is obtained. When iodized oil is used, another film is obtained in twenty-four hours to detect the extent of the overflow into the peivis through the uterine tubes.

Radiographic Appearance (Fig. 11.8)

Hysterosalpingogram

Uterine tubes appear as passing from the upper angles of the uterus and taking a tortuous course laterally. The calibre is less in the medial two-thirds, but is wider at the ovarian ends.

Peritoneal spill of the contrast medium is a sign of patency of the fallopian tube.

Uterus cavity shadow appears triangular with the apex towards the pelvis.

PELVIMETRY

Direct Radiography of Female Pelvis (Fig. 11.9)

It is resorted to assess the configuration of the maternal pelvis as well as the age of the foetus. In any case, radiation exposure of the patient and the foetus in the first trimester of pregnancy is to be avoided unless and until very necessary. The following criteria are used in giving an opinion as to the maturity of the foetus.

An ossification centre is present in the lower end of the femur in 90 per cent of full-term foetuses; ossification of the hyoid bone is complete, and five out of six cases will show ossification in the upper tibial epiphysis. Less practical standards

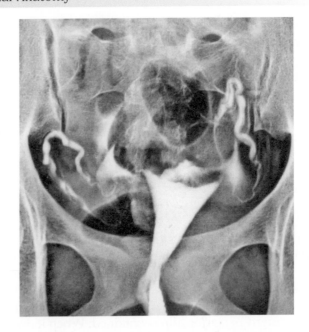

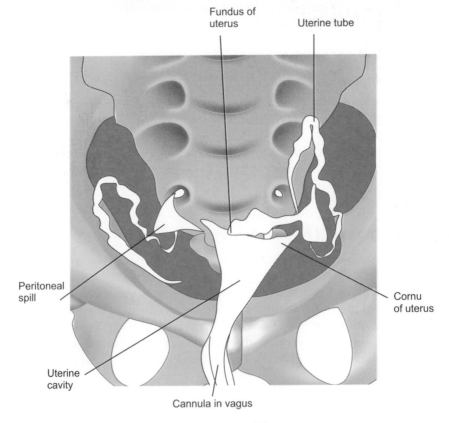

Fig. 11.8: Uretrus—hysterosalpingogram

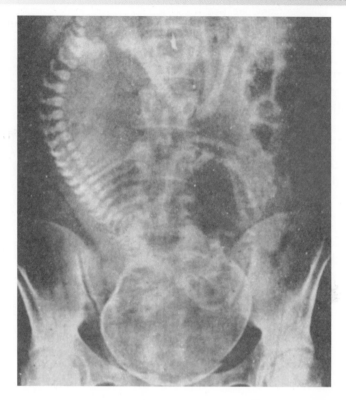

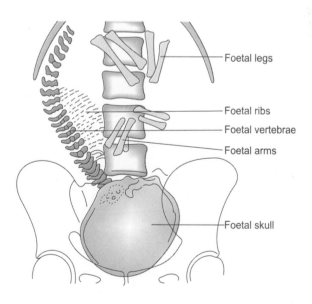

Foetal legs

Foetal ribs

Foetal vertebrae

Foetal arms

Foetal skull

Fig. 11.9: Pregnant uterus—foetal parts

are the ossification of the essential parts of vertebrae, the first segment of the coccyx, and the metacarpals and phalanges.

The other information which can be gained is:

- Presentation and position of the foetus
- Degree of flexion of the foetal head and spine
- Viability of foetus
- Progress of labour
- Diagnosis of multiple pregnancy
- Detection of the early foetus
- Position of the placenta.

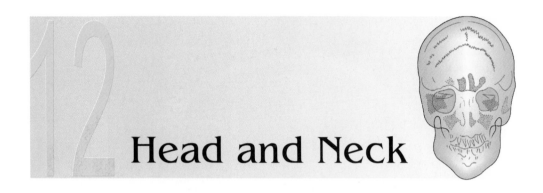

Head and Neck

SKULL

RADIOGRAPHIC APPEARANCE

Lateral View (Fig. 12.1)

- **Anterior clinoid process** points posteriorly over the pituitary fossa.
- **Anterior cranial fossa** is a distinct white line passing posteriorly from near the base of the frontal sinus to the anterior clinoid process.
- **Coronal suture** extends as a *zigzag* translucent line from the vertex for a variable distance.
- **External ear** margins may cast shadows above the petrous part of the temporal bone.
- **External and internal auditory meatus** of both sides cast a 5 mm ring shadow near the centre of the triangle of petrous temporal.
- **Frontal sinus** appears as triangular translucent area with the base downwards and situated at the base of the frontal bone anteriorly.
- **Hard palate and teeth** are situated below the maxillary sinus.
- **Lambdoid suture** extends downwards and forwards from the posterior part of the vault of skull to the base just behind the dense triangular shadow of the petrous temporal.
- **Mastoid air cells** appear as honeycomb translucencies lying behind the ring of external auditary meatus.
- **Maxillary sinus** is seen below the orbit as a translucent area.
- **Middle meningeal groove** is seen as a dark arborising line starting in the region of sella turcica situated 1 cm behind the line of the coronal suture and ascending towards the top of the vault. A smaller and less prominent vascular groove due to the posterior division of the meningeal vessels is often seen branching off the main groove just above the base of the skull and posteriorly and slightly upwards.

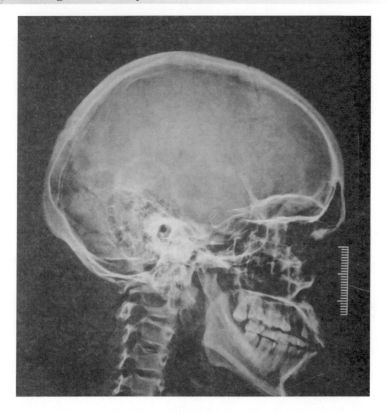

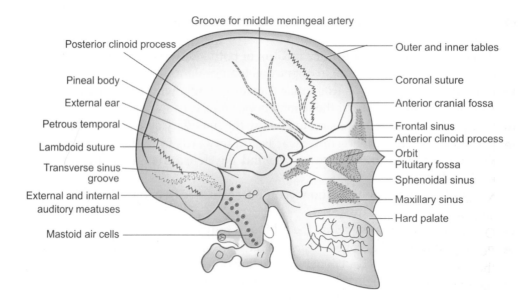

Fig. 12.1: Skull—lateral view

Groove for middle meningeal artery
Posterior clinoid process
Outer and inner tables
Pineal body
Coronal suture
External ear
Anterior cranial fossa
Petrous temporal
Frontal sinus
Anterior clinoid process
Lambdoid suture
Orbit
Transverse sinus groove
Pituitary fossa
Sphenoidal sinus
External and internal auditory meatuses
Maxillary sinus
Hard palate
Mastoid air cells

- **Orbit** casts a shadow in front of the ethmoidal sinuses.
- **Outer and inner tables** appear as dense white lines separated by dipole.
- **Petrous temporal** casts a dense triangular shadow with upper margin horizontal and posterior margin running almost vertically downwards.
- **Pineal body** casts a small shadow above and behind the external auditory meatus after early adult life when it is calcified.
- **Pituitary fossa** is seen as a round or oval depression resting on the sphenoidal air sinuses.

Radiographs of the sella turcica may reveal minor abnormalities which are easily overlooked at a cursory examination, but since they may precede definite clinical evidence of serious disease it is most important that a careful study of the region should be made. The abnormalities may be:

    a. Erosion due to raised intracranial pressure,
    b. Ballooning due to pituitary tumour,
    c. Non-specific enlargement,
    d. Flattening due to suprasellar space occupying lesions.

- **Posterior clinoid process** is seen projecting from each side of the upper margin of the dorsum sellae.
- **Sphenoidal sinuses** are seen as translucent shadows below and anterior to the hypophyseal fossa.
- **Transverse sinus groove** appears as a translucent curved band-like shadow about 1 cm wide behind the petrous temporal area.

Antero-Posterior View (Fig. 12.2)

- **Coronal suture** meets the sagittal suture near the vertex.
- **Frontal sinuses** appear as translucent areas above and between the orbits.
- **Greater wing of sphenoid,** its lateral edge is represented by a white line which descends from the lateral part of the line representing the lesser wing. This line descends downwards and medially across the lateral third of the orbit.
- **Lambdoid suture** is seen a little below the coronal suture.
- **Lesser wing of sphenoid** is seen as a white line extenting across the orbital shadow.
- **Mandibular condyles** can be traced down to the more obvious ramus of mandible.
- **Mastoid process and mastoid air cells** are visible laterally and inferiorly.
- **Maxillary sinuses** lie adjacent to the inferior margin of the orbit and the petrous temporal shadow is superimposed.
- **Nasal fossae** are seen on each side of the nasal septum. Sphenoidal and ethmoidal sinuses are superimposed.
- **Orbits** are seen distinctly below and lateral to the frontal sinuses.
- **Petrous temporal** forms a dense white shadow running directly medially across the orbit and the maxillary air sinus.
- **Sagittal suture** is seen placed centrally.

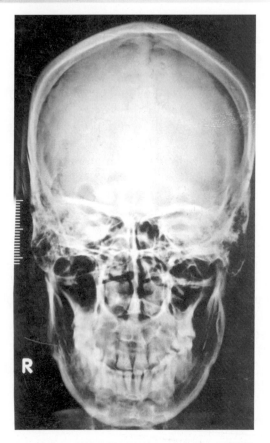

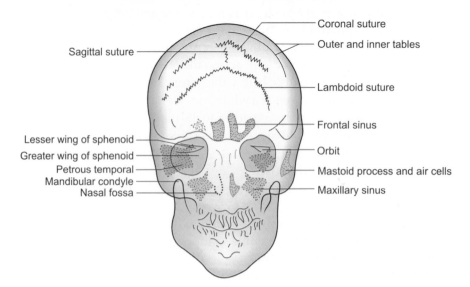

Fig. 12.2: Skull—antero-posterior view

Posterior-Anterior (Caldwell) View (Fig. 12.3)

This view shows para-nasal air sinuses clearly. Other features of the skull can also
be made out.

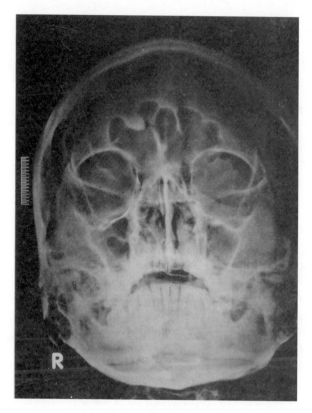

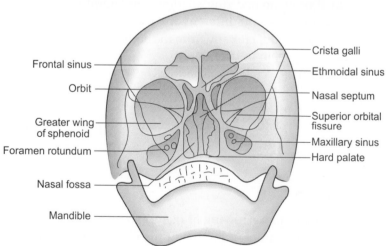

Frontal sinus

Orbit

Greater wing
of sphenoid

Foramen rotundum

Nasal fossa

Mandible

Crista galli

Ethmoidal sinus

Nasal septum

Superior orbital
fissure

Maxillary sinus

Hard palate

Fig. 12.3: Skull—Caldwell view

Vertebral Column $\big|$ 13

RADIOGRAPHIC APPEARANCE

ANTERO-POSTERIOR AND LATERAL VIEWS

General Features (Figs 13.5 and 13.6)

- **Articular facets** are imperfectly seen.
- **Intervertebral discs** are seen as translucent intervals between the bodies.
- **Laminae** can be seen partly overlapping the intervertebral spaces and partly the vertebral bodies in antero-posterior view.
- **Pedicles** are fore-shortened in antero-posterior view and appear as ring-shaped shadows on the lateral parts of the bodies. In a lateral view they are seen projecting backwards.
- **Spinous processes** in the antero-posterior view are fore-shortened and appear as centrally placed oval or elongated ring shadows, in lateral view they are seen clearly projecting backwards with different obliquity.
- **Transverse processes** stand out laterally from the bodies in antero-posterior view but are superimposed on them in lateral view.
- **Vertebral bodies** appear as rectangular shadows.

SPECIAL FEATURES

CERVICAL SPINE

Antero-posterior View (Fig. 13.1)

- **Larynx** appears as an abrupt narrowing at the upper end of trachea.
- **Mandible** shadow is superimposed on that of the upper cervical vertebrae.
- **Thyroid cartilage** shadow is seen opposite the bodies of cervical fourth and fifth vertebrae.

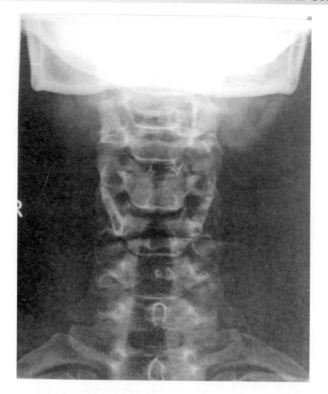

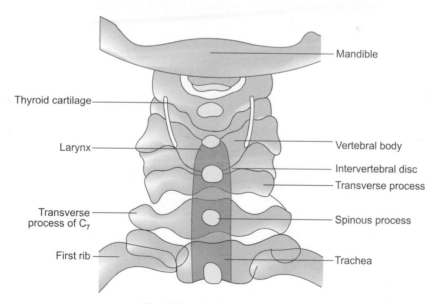

Mandible

Thyroid cartilage

Larynx

Vertebral body

Intervertebral disc

Transverse process

Transverse process of C₇

Spinous process

First rib

Trachea

Fig. 13.1: Cervical spine—AP view

- **Trachea** is seen as a centrally placed tubular translucency in the cervical and upper thoracic regions.
- **Transverse process of** C7 points downwards and laterally in contrast to the transverse process of first thoracic vertebra which is inclined upwards and laterally. This distinction is valuable in cases of cervical rib which might otherwise cause confusion.

LATERAL VIEW (Fig. 13.2)

- **Anterior arch of atlas** shadow is seen in front of the odontoid process.
- **Odontoid process** is seen as an upward extension from the body of cervical second.
- **Pedicles** from the cervical third downwards cast a circular or oval shadow on the bodies of the vertebrae.
- **Spines of the 2nd, 3rd and 4th cervical** are sometimes befid; the spine of cervical seventh is the longest.

 ## THORACIC SPINE

ANTERO-POSTERIOR VIEW (Fig. 13.3)

- **Joint spaces** are imperfectly seen.
- **Spinous processes** appear as centrally placed oval or elongated ring shadows.
- **Transverse processes** are obscured by the ribs.

LATERAL VIEW (Fig. 13.4)

- **Spines and neural arches** are obscured by the overlying rib shadows.
- **Vertebral bodies of upper thoracic** are often obscured by the shoulder girdle.

 ## LUMBAR SPINE

ANTERO-POSTEIOR VIEW (Fig. 13.5)

- **Intervertebral joints** appear as nearly horizontal slits close above or overlapping the outlines of the pedicles.
- **Neural arches** partly overlap the intervertebral spaces and partly overlap the vertebral bodies.

LATERAL VIEW (Fig. 13.6)

A line drawn along the posterior border of the body of sacrum and the posterior borders of the bodies of the lumbar vertebrae, may be expected to form an even curve.

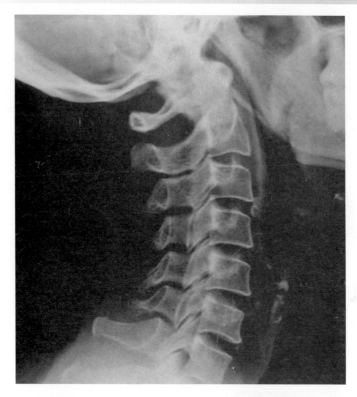

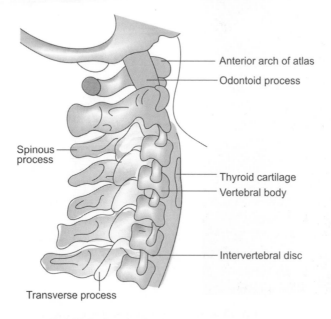

Fig. 13.2: Cervical spine—lateral view

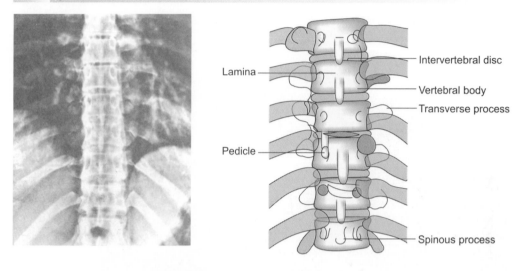

Fig. 13.3: Thoracic spine—AP view

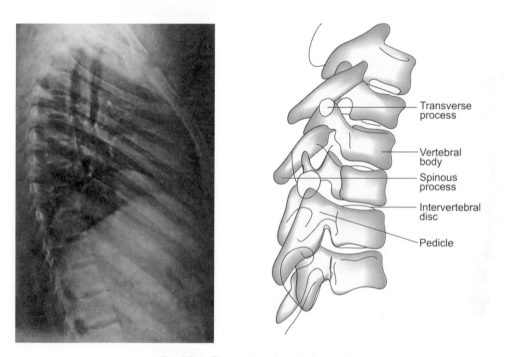

Fig. 13.4: Thoracic spine—lateral view

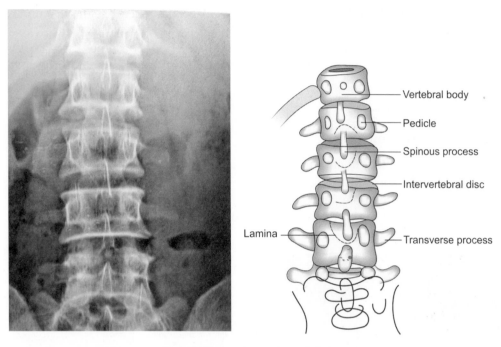

Fig. 13.5: Lumbar spine—AP view

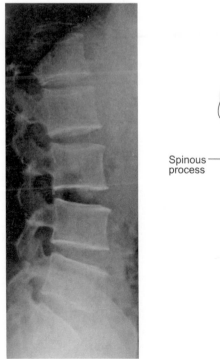

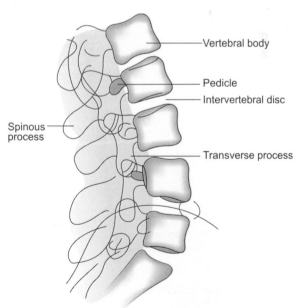

Fig. 13.6: Lumbar spine—lateral view

- **Lumbarisation of first sacral segment.** When the first sacral segment fails to fuse, it is termed as the sixth lumbar vertebra.
- **Sacralisation of lumbar vertebra.** The 5th lumbar vertebra becomes fused partly or completely with the first sacral segment and then there are only four lumbar vertebrae.

SACRUM AND COCCYX

Antero-posterior View (Figs 13.7a and b)

- **Coccyx** varies in length and may not be exactly in the midline.
- **Sacral foramina** are clearly seen.
- **Sacroiliac joint.** Double joint lines are seen, the lateral one corresponds to the anterior edge and the medial one to the posterior edge of the sacroiliac joint.

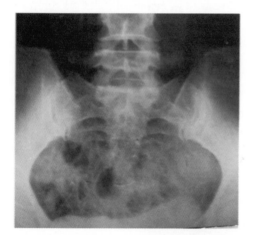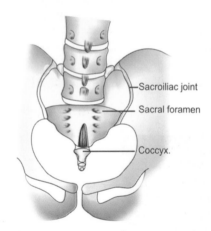

Fig. 13.7a: Sacrum and coccyx—AP view

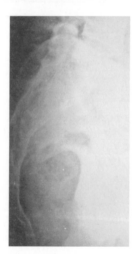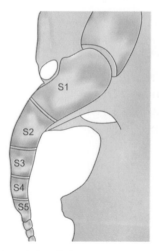

Fig. 13.7b: Sacrum and coccyx—lateral view

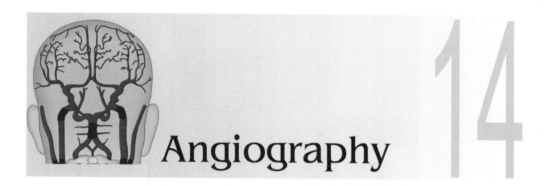

Angiography

Angiography is a roentgenologic procedure which permits visualisation of the internal anatomy of the heart and blood vessels including arteries, veins and lymphatics through the intravascular injection of radiopaque contrast material. Indications are many and varied.

CONTRAST MEDIA

The ideal contrast medium should possess three qualities:
  i. high specificity and radiopacity.
 ii. low toxicity.
iii. low viscosity.

None of the available media reach the ideal. The commonly available media in our country are Conray, Visotrast, Diaginol and Urographin in concentrations of 50% and 75%. The usual dose of these is between 20 and 60 ml varying according to the age, height, body weight, and volume of vascular bed to be visualised.

Abdominal aortography and cerebral arteriography will be coinsidered as examples.

AORTOGRAPHY (Fig . 14.1)

Through aortography one may obtain a visualisation of the entire aortic circulation and its branches. It is also useful for visualisation of the placenta in the pregnant uterus. Since there is a pudding of dye in the sinusoidal circulation of the placenta it is readily visualised and abnormal implantation can be detected.

Its greatest use lies in the demonstration of renal architecture. A wide variety of pathologic conditions of the kidney such as neoplasms, anomalies, aneurysms and causes of renal hypertension can be diagnosed.

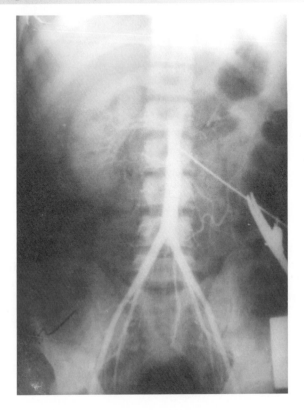

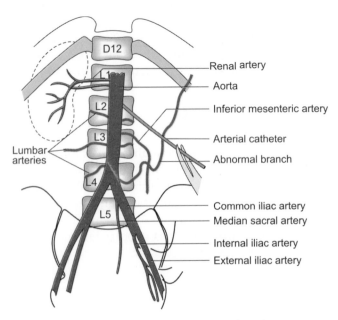

Fig. 14.1: Aortogram—abdominal aorta

Two commonly used techniques of abdominal aortography are:
  i. **Translumbar aortography.** Direct needle puncture of the vessel
      - The needle is introduced through the skin just below the 12th rib about 5 cm on the left of the midline. It is directed anteriorly, upwards and medially till it grazes against the lateral surface of the vertebral body. It is then withdrawn a little and readjusted till the transmitted pulsations of the aorta are felt. Additional pressure forces it into the lumen, which is indicated by the gush of blood into the tubing.
      - By a 10 ml syringe 5 ml of the medium is injected and the position of the needle is checked by screening or an X-ray, following this 40 ml medium is injected forcefully by a 50 ml syringe in shortest possible time.
 ii. **Retrograde transfemoral aortography (Modified Seldinger's method)**
      - The patient is put in the supine position and the femoral arteries are felt on both sides. The one with better pulsation is preferred and the inguinal area is prepared and draped.
      - A small skin incision is made over the pulsating artery. The artery is punctured with a Seldinger's needle No. 18 gauge with double lumen and bevelled edges, till a free blood flow is obtained.
      - A flexible guide wire is introduced into the arterial lumen and the needle is withdrawn.
      - An arterial catheter of Odman's type is slipped down over the guide wire into the artery and is advanced into the aorta up to the desired level. Fluoroscopic help is safe and beneficial at this stage.
      - The guide wire is then removed leaving the catheter in the artery.
      - Rest of the steps are the same as in the translumbar technique.

The advantage of catheter method over direct needle puncture is that with the catheter in position the bolus of the dye can be injected at selected levels and the injection of the dye can be repeated at intervals if necessary.

CEREBRAL ANGIOGRAPHY (Figs 14.2a and b)

Carotid Angiography

Carotid angiography is done to visualise lesions above the tentorium cerebelli particularly those in the anterior two-thirds of the hemisphere.

Techniques

A Cournands needle of 18 gauge is used for puncturing the common carotid artery.

The skin up to the outer carotid wall is punctured with a sharp stylet in position while the needle is threaded in the artery with a blunt stylet.
  - The sharp stylet is taken out when the artery gets punctured. The needle is gradually withdrawn to get a jet of arterial blood through the spout of the needle.

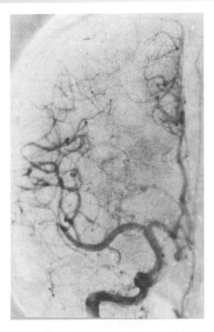

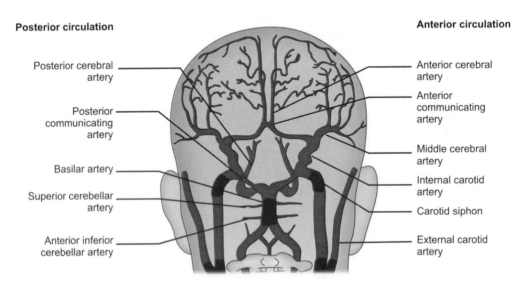

Posterior circulation

Posterior cerebral artery

Posterior communicating artery

Basilar artery

Superior cerebellar artery

Anterior inferior cerebellar artery

Anterior circulation

Anterior cerebral artery

Anterior communicating artery

Middle cerebral artery

Internal carotid artery

Carotid siphon

External carotid artery

Fig. 14.2a: Antero-posterior internal carotid angiogram

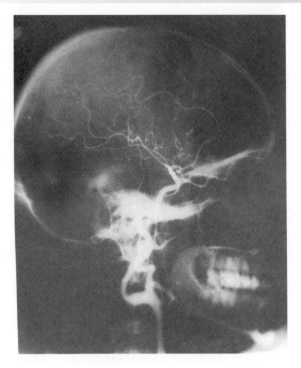

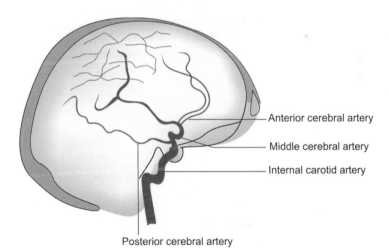

Anterior cerebral artery

Middle cerebral artery

Internal carotid artery

Posterior cerebral artery

Fig. 14.2b: Angiogram-Internal carotid artery—lateral view

- The syringe is next filled up with 10 ml of the contrast medium. The contrast dye used is Urografin 75% or Conrary 280 or Visotrast 370. The latter two have approximate concentration of 60%. The dye is injected fairly rapidly with a considerable force.
- The first picture is shot as the last 2 ml of contrast medium is left to be injected. The next two pictures are taken at 1½ and 2 seconds, after complete injection of dye respectively.
- Both the antero-posterior and lateral projections should be taken whenever possible, since only then can one consider the visualisation complete in three dimensions.

VERTEBRAL ANGIOGRAPHY (Fig. 14.3)

It is done to visualise lesions below the tentorium cerebelli. The technique of vertebral puncture is almost the same through the neck as for the carotid artery puncture described above.

- The needle is held almost vertical (perpendicular) to neck and is inserted up to the transverse process of the seventh cervical vertebra.
- After the above structure is struck, the needle is withdrawn and inserted with a slight inclination of 45° or 50°.

There is another technique of obtaining a vertebral angiogram, i.e. via right brachial route.

- A percutaneous puncture of right brachial artery is done 3.75 cm above its division (and about the same distance from the crease of right elbow joint).

The amount of dye used is greater than in carotid angiography. In one view 30 ml of contrast medium is used in the same concentration as that for carotid angiography.

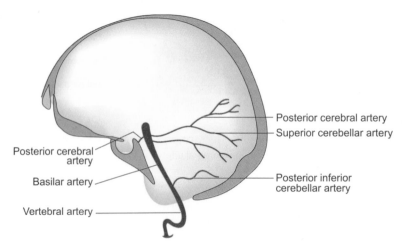

Fig. 14.3: Angiogram-Vertebral artery—lateral view

New Imaging Devices

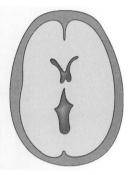

A new breed of computerized body-scanning devices is changing the face of medicine. Recent rapid advances in imaging technology or "machine vision"enable doctors to see inside the body without exploratory operations. The technology of computer graphics is being harnessed to transform the torrents of "machine vision" data into meaningful diagnostic displays. As a result more progress has been made in diagnostic medicine in the past fifteen years than in the entire previous history of medicine.

1. COMPUTED TOMOGRAPHY (CT) (Figs 15.1 to 15.8)

The technique was developed in Great Britain in 1972. It employs an X-ray tube on a yoke that allows 360 degrees rotation. A thin fan-shaped X-ray beam penetrates the body and produces a cross-sectional view of tissues within. By revolving the X-ray tube around the body, CT machines view thin "Slices" of the body from many angles. Hundreds of crystal chip detectors move in an arc with the X-ray tube. The detectors on the opposite side of the tube record what the scanner sees and deliver their information to a digital computer which compares the many views to make a single three-dimensional video image which is displayed on a screen.

Thus CT scan is a cross-sectional image presented as a matrix of picture elements or pixels. Each pixel records on a grey scale the X-ray absorption of the corresponding element in the patient and, since these absorption values vary in a systematic way from tissue to tissue, this process builds up a picture of the organs and tissues.

CT scan has profound use in lesions of the brain and spinal cord. Though expensive, it is a non-invasive, quick method to evaluate patients for brain, spinal cord and vertebral column lesions.

Haematomas, infective lesions of the brain, cerebrovascular accidents whether due to infarct or haemorrhage can be differentiated easily. Mass whether supratentorial or infratentorial can be better evaluated using plain contrast enhanced scans. Ventricular system enlargement or diplacement can be easily recognised. Lesions around the sella turcica and other extra-axial tumours can be confidently diagnosed.

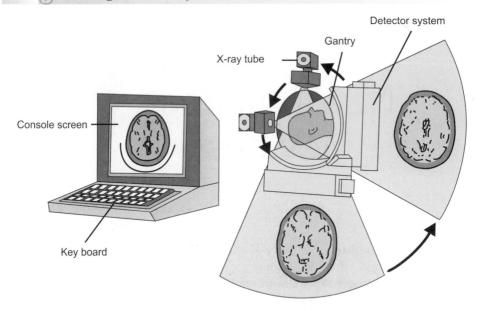

Fig. 15.1: CT technique

In the spinal cord, tumours can be seen using myelogram followed by CT scan. The lesions of the vertebral column like infections, tumours, congenital abnormalities in the cranio-vertebral regions, disc prolapse, spondylolisthesis, etc. can be clearly seen.

In the nasopharynx, oropharynx and larynx it has a significant diagnostic role. Lesions of the orbit, lymph nodes, thyroid and parathyroid glands, salivary glands can be seen clearly.

CT images have a number of advantages over conventional chest radiographs, for example the absence of confusing superimposition of structures and superior contrast resolution. CT scanning has a limited place in cardiology because the movements of the heart and the relatively long scanning time make the images too blurred to be of value. In thorax parenchymal and mediastinal masses can be seen clearly.

CT scans are valuable to demonstrate focal or diffuse, solid or cystic lesions in the liver. Masses of the gallbladder and their extension in the liver is better seen. Lesions in the pancreas can be diagnosed confidently. Lymph node and splenic enlargements can be clearly seen in properly done studies.

CT scanning has a major role in diseases of the hollow viscera. Barium meal and endoscopic examinations remain the investigation of choice for the gastro-intestinal tract. Scanning methods do, however, provide additional valuable information in certain circumstances.

Since CT scans display anatomy in the axial plane the technique has become important in the demonstration of urinary tract abnormalities. Radiologically non-opaque calculi (composed of xanthine, uric acid or cystine) have a high density on

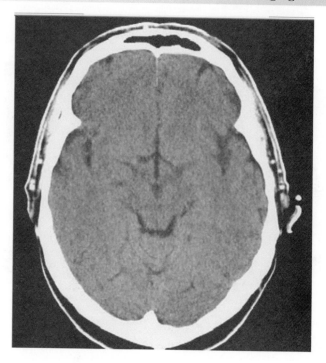

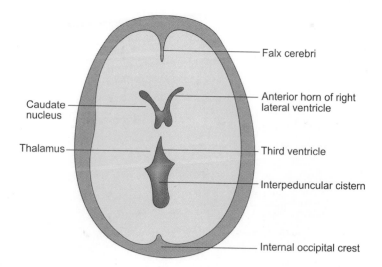

Fig. 15.2: CT scan brain at the level of interpeduncular cistern

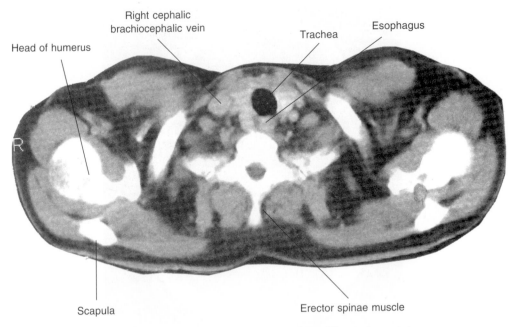

Fig. 15.3: CT scan thorax at the level of third thoracic vertebra

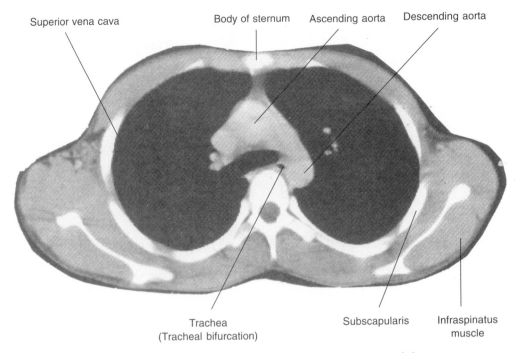

Fig. 15.4: CT scan thorax at the level of fourth thoracic vertebra

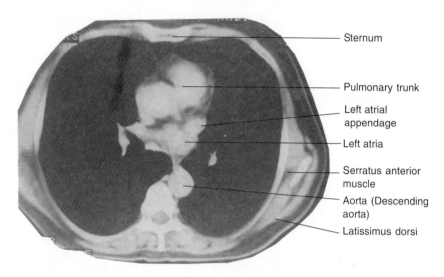

Sternum

Pulmonary trunk

Left atrial appendage

Left atria

Serratus anterior muscle

Aorta (Descending aorta)

Latissimus dorsi

Fig. 15.5: CT scan thorax at the level of fifth thoracic vertebra

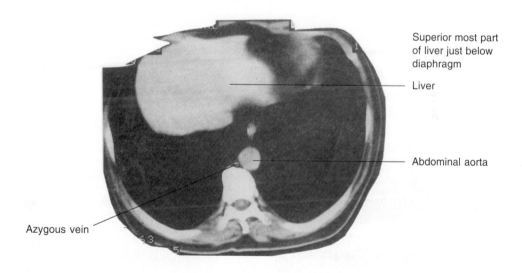

Superior most part of liver just below diaphragm

Liver

Abdominal aorta

Azygous vein

Fig. 15.6: CT scan thorax at the level of eleventh thoracic vertebra

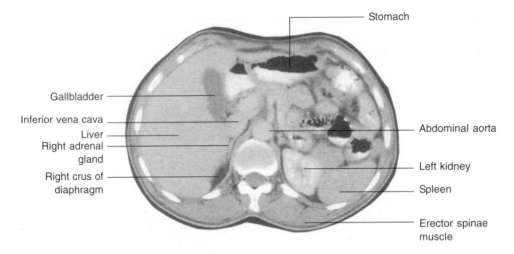

Fig. 15.7: CT scan abdomen at the level of twelfth thoracic vertebra

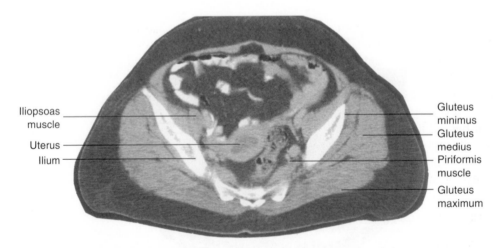

Fig. 15.8: CT scan pelvis at the level of third sacral vertebra

CT scanning and can be distinguished from other caliceal filling defects, such as blood clots and small tumours.

In the pelvis, urinary bladder, prostate, seminal vesicles, uterus and ovaries can be imaged and their lesions detected.

2. MAGNETIC RESONANCE IMAGING (MRI) (Figs 15.9 and 15.10)

Instead of X-rays a combination of radio-waves and a strong magnetic field are used in this revolutionary technique. It relies on the principle that hydrogen atoms when subjected to a magnetic field line up. If a radio-frequency is aimed at these atoms, it changes the alignment of their nuclei. When the radio-waves are turned off, the nuclei realign themselves, transmitting a small electrical signal. Since the body is primarily composed of hydrogen atoms, an image can be generated from the returning pulses, showing tissue and bone marrow as never seen before. The tissues having higher water density appear brightest with MRI since it focuses on the behaviour of hydrogen atoms in water molecule. This allows MRI to do certain things better than CT scanners, such as distinguishing between the brains white matter and water rich grey matter. Teeth and bones which contains little water, do not appear at all in MRI, enabling doctors to see tissues surrounded by bone, such as the spinal cord.

The contrast resolution of MRI is superior to that of CT scanning and cross-sectional images can be obtained in any plane. It is being increasingly used for imaging the heart and great vessels as it can distinguish between tissues better than CT scanning and can identify structures containing flowing blood.

MRI has proved to be an effective means of examining the spinal cord because of its ability to depict soft tissues in high contrast. Examination of spinal cord with X-ray required injection of a contrast medium during a procedure which could be risky and painful.

It has limitations in calcified structures because they contain very small amount of water which is the source for hydrogen ions. CT scan is better than MRI in the lesion of such structures. An additional advantage of MRI is that it involves no X-ray radiation.

3. ULTRASONOGRAPHY (Figs 15.11 to 15.14)

It uses sound waves to look within. A small transducer or transmitter receiver is placed in contact with the area of the body being investigated. High frequency sound waves penetrate the body, strike the organs within, and reflect back to the surface, where the transducer now functions as a receiver. The time delays of these returning signals sketch the targets location, size, shape, even its texture, for a display line by line on a screen. Echoes are thus translated into faint signals which are processed by computer into a video image.

Rapid anatomic 'real time' or two dimensional scanning allows clear visualisation of tissue movements which assist in the identification of anatomical and pathological structures. It is a non-invasive rapid and safe technique and gives good details. The accuracy of ultrasound diagnosis is 90%.

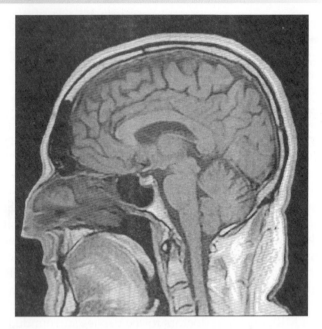

Fig. 15.9: Midline sagittal magnetic resonance image (MRI) of normal brain

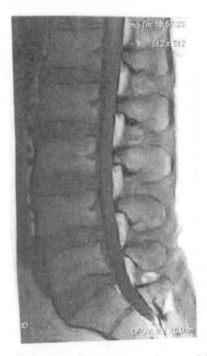

Fig. 15.10: Midline sagittal magnetic resonance image (MRI) of normal spinal cord

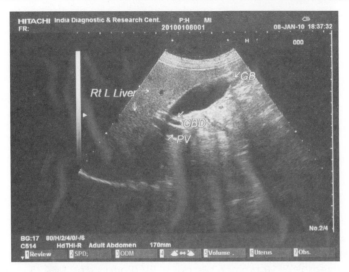

Fig. 15.11: USG through gallbladder GB (Gallbladder), CBD (Common bile duct), PV (Portal vein)

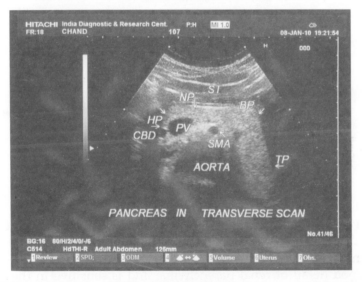

Fig. 15.12: USG through pancreas ST (Stomach), NP (Neck of pancreas), BP (body of pancreas), HP (head of pancreas), CBD (common bile duct), PV (Portal vein), SMA (Superior mesenteric artery), TP (Tail of pancreas)

Solid and cystic structures transmit sound waves in straight lines, and reflect them from interfaces. Gas filled structures dissipate the ultrasonic beam, and therefore the liver, gallbladder and solid or cystic tumours in the abdomen can be depicted by abdominal ultrasound. Structures which reflect ultrasound appear bright (hyperechoic), whereas structures which transmit ultrasound appear dark (hypoechoic).

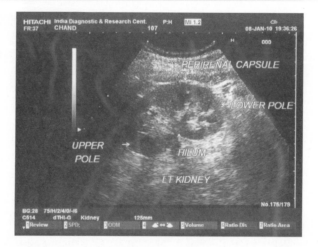

Fig. 15.13: USG through pancreas ST (Stomach), NP (Neck of pancreas), BP (body of pancreas), HP (head of pancreas), CBD (common bile duct), PV (Portal vein), SMA (Superior mesenteric artery), TP (Tail of pancreas)

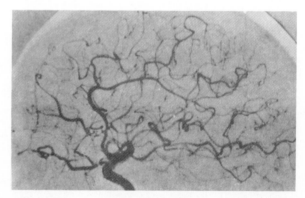

Fig. 15.14: Digital subtraction angiography of cerebral vessels

The most significant application of ultrasound has been in the diagnosis of gallbladder disease, the differential diagnosis of jaundice and diseases of liver. It is cheaper than CT scanning.

It gives good detail of renal parenchyma, and is sensitive in the detection of hydronephrosis, non-opaque stones and perirenal collections. The normal ureter is not routinely visualised, but is seen when dilated. The mid-section of the ureter is often obscured by overlying structures particularly gas containing bowel, but the lower ureter should easily be seen in filled bladder. Bladder abnormalities may be identified, the size of the prostate may be assessed, and bladder volume before and after voiding can be measured.

It is the only body scanning technique recommended for pregnant women, and has tremendous application in diagnosing the diseases of uterus and ovaries. In pregnancy it is being widely used for age and sex determination, congenital anomalies of foetus, placental abnormalities and to see the presentation of the foetus.

The viability and growth of the foetus are monitored periodically by ultrasound. In case of infertility it is useful for timing the follicular maturation which helps in many ways. Ultrasound has useful applications for diseases of thyroid and parathyroids, breast, neonatal head, orbit and scrotum.

Ultrasonography of heart is known as **Echocardiography.** Two echocardiographic methods are in use at the present time, the M-Mode and the cross-sectional, otherwise known as 'real time' or two dimensional. The M-Mode records the echoes of structures along a single linear beam emanating from a transducer placed on the precordium. From this the movement of the right and left ventricular cavity and wall thickness can be measured as well as the movement of the mitral, aortic and tricuspid valves. The pulmonary valve is less readily echoed. Echocardiography is one of the certain ways of diagnosing prolapsed mitral cusps. In cross-sectional echocardiography the images obtained from the two-dimensional echo are dynamic so that movement of the ventricles can be seen directly, as well as the functioning of the valves.

Echocardiography has a very important place in congenital heart disease. The interatrial and interventricular septa are relatively easy to visualise and the presence of a defect in either of these can almost always be seen if they are of a size which is clinically significant.

4. DIGITAL SUBTRACTION ANGIOGRAPHY (DSA)

It is an imaging technique that produces clean clear views of flowing blood or its blockage by narrowed vessels. DSA depends on the injection into the vessels of a contrast agent containing iodine that is opaque to X-rays. The shadow, this opacity creats allow doctors to see the flow of blood. Before injection of the contrast substance, an X-ray image is made and stored in a computer. After injection a second image is made highlighting the flowing blood as revealed by the substance. The computer then substracts image one from image two, leaving a sharp picture of blood vessels such as the coronary arteries. It is thus a method for computerised enchancement of the images obtained at angiography.

5. RADIO-ISOTOPE IMAGING (PET/SPECT)

Positron emission tomography (PET) and single photon emission computed tomography (SPECT) are a form of radio-isotope imaging. SPECT shows blood flow by imaging trace amounts of radio-isotopes. PET can also measure metabolism revealing how well the body is working. The use of radioactive tracers is well suited to studies of epilepsy, schizophrenia, Parkinson's disease and can indicate brain damage from a stroke.

Both PET and SPECT depict the distribution of blood into tissue, but PET does so with greater accuracy. By tracing the radioactive substance, a doctor can pin point areas of abnormal brain activity or determine the health of cells.

Index